The Nightingale Sisters

The Making of a Nurse in 1800's America

Compiled

By Rosalind Franklin

'Make your Daughters Independent' by C Andreas originally published in 'The Century Magazine; a popular quarterly' Volume 36, Issue 1, May 1885

'A New Profession for Women' by Franklin D North, originally published in 'The Century Magazine' November 1882

'The Connecticut Training School for Nurses' by Anon, originally published in 'The Century' Volume 30, Issue 6, October 1885

'The Training of a Nurse' Mary Cadwalader Jones, originally published in Scribner's Magazine, Volume 8, Issue 5, November 1890

'A Nurse Should be' originally published in 'Ambulance Work And Nursing: A Handbook On First Aid To The Injured' W. T. Keener & Co. Chicago, 1895

'A Great Charity Reform' by E V Smalley originally published in 'The Century' Volume 24, Issue 3, July 1882

British Library Cataloguing In Publication Data
A Record of This Publication is available from the British Library

ISBN 0-9515655-8-3

This edition first published April 2005 by Diggory Press, an imprint of Meadow Books, 35 Stonefield Way, Burgess Hill, West Sussex, RH15 8DW, UK
Email: meadowbooks@hotmail.com or visit www.diggorypress.com

INDEX

CHAPTER ONE

Make Your Daughters Independent

It is the refinement of cruelty to educate girls in the aimless fashion of today. Boys are trained to look forward to a career of usefulness while girls grow up without any fixed purpose in life, unless indeed their hopes and ambitions center upon marriage, as is most often the case.

While it is natural and right for girls to look forward to marriage, it will be well for them all when they fully appreciate the undeniable fact that marriage is a remoter possibility now than it was in the days of their grandmothers, and that even those whose fondest dreams may one day be realized have much to do and to learn before they are ready for the life upon which they will enter with such high and happy hopes.

No woman is qualified for marriage until she understands domestic economy in all its branches; the management of servants and the care of the sick arid children; is proficient in needlework; and besides all this possesses a thorough knowledge of some business, profession, trade, or calling which will insure her independence on occasion. Now, as a rule, none of these things are taught in school.

It is obvious, therefore, that if they are to be learned it must he done after school life is over. How often one hears a married woman, the mother of a young family who would look to her for support if suddenly deprived of their natural protector, deplore her ignorance of any one accomplishment that would afford her a competence. It is not too much to say that such a one bad no right to marry. It was assuming too great a risk; for no more cruel fate can befall a woman than to be cast upon a cold and heartless world without the means of earning a livelihood for herself and those who may be dependent upon her.

A time is liable to come in every life when the all-important question will arise, 'What can I do to make money?' The possession of wealth is one of the most uncertain things in life, especially in this country. On the other side of the water, where estates remain in the same family from one generation to another, there is more stability in riches. But here a man may be rich today, poor tomorrow, and in a few short months or years his children may see want: witness the series of financial crashes that have lately visited this country.

There is many a one suffering today for the common necessaries of life whose future seemed radiant with the light of assured prosperity when the New Year dawned. Upon none does the weight of such sore trials fall more heavily than upon the women who, having been reared in the lap of luxury, are thus suddenly forced by cruel necessity to turn their attention to something that will keep the wolf from the door. But why did they not anticipate misfortune and make provision for it in more prosperous days? Simply because they had not the courage to defy public opinion.

There is a class of women who need more sympathy and get less than their share. They are those who in girlhood, through no fault of their own, led the listless, aimless life already described, but who in late years, by some untoward circumstance, are brought face to face with the sad realities of life. Cultured, refined women, who have seen better days, find the struggle for life far more hitter than their more fortunate sisters whose position in life has always been such as to necessitate their earning their own livings. It is for such this plea is made.

Domestic servants are well off in America; they are the most independent class of women-workers. The great army of shop girls, factory girls, sewing girls, those engaged in trades of all kinds, may congratulate themselves upon their comparatively happy lot. They often look with envy upon those who, they fancy, are better off than themselves. Let them cultivate a spirit of contentment.

There are trials - bitter, bitter trials - in the lives of some of those they are foolish enough to envy, of which they know nothing. There are miseries of which they never dream. An accomplished lady, daughter of an army officer who some score or more of years ago served his country nobly in her hour of peril, is today learning the art of telegraphy in one of our Western cities, in the hope that she may be enabled thereby to support her little children. In the happy home of her youth, no expense was spared upon this lady's education. She was exceptionally talented and won an enviable reputation as a skillful pianist. It was not surprising that this petted favorite of fortune contracted a brilliant marriage.

Her pathway seemed strewn with roses, and for years not a cloud of care or sorrow shadowed her young life. But trouble came at last. Death robbed her, at one stroke, of her noble husband and a much loved child. Then financial troubles followed, and in a few short months this delicately nurtured gentlewoman found herself bereft of fortune also. Grief-stricken as she was, she felt that there was something still left to live for; and, for the sake of her two little ones, she took up the burden of life and faced the future bravely. Naturally she thought her knowledge of music would afford her the needed means of support. But, alas, she soon found that accomplishments are of small avail in the struggle for a living, and that teaching music was too precarious a means of earning money to be depended upon with any degree of certainty for the support of a family.

Although so costly a thing to acquire, an education cannot always be made to yield proper returns for the time and money expended upon it. The bitter truth soon forced itself upon this unfortunate woman's mind that a servant in anybody's kitchen was better off, financially, than she. She must therefore learn something at once that will be of more marketable value than the accomplishments of which, until now, she has all her life been justly proud.

7

Hence we find her laboring to master a new and difficult art at an age when study is not an easy matter. Her children, meanwhile, are being cared for by kind friends. Would it not be wiser far to induce young girls in thousands of happy, prosperous homes to make ample provision for any and all emergencies that the future may have in store for them? Could a better use be found for some of the years that intervene between the time a girl leaves school and the time she may reasonably hope to marry? The field for woman's work has been opened up of late years in so many different directions that a vocation can easily be found, outside the profession of teaching that will be quite as congenial to refined tastes, and considerably more lucrative. Book-keeping, typewriting, telegraphy, stenography, engraving, dentistry, medicine, nursing, and a dozen other occupations might be mentioned.

Then, too, industrial schools might he established, where the daughters of wealthy parents could be trained in the practical details of any particular industry for which they displayed a special aptitude. If it is not beneath the sons and daughters of a monarch to learn a trade, it ought not to be beneath the sons and daughters of republican America to emulate their good example, provided they possess the requisite ability to do so. Two years will suffice to make any bright, quick girl conversant with all the mysteries of the art of housekeeping, especially if she be wise enough to study the art practically as well as theoretically.

The management of servants and the care of the sick and children will be incidentally learned in most homes, and can be supplemented by a more extended study of physiology, hygiene, etc. than was possible at school. Sewing need not be neglected either, while leisure will readily be found for reading or any other recreation that may suit individual tastes. Another year, or longer, may be added to the time devoted to these pursuits, if desired. But, above all, let two or three years be conscientiously set apart for the express purpose of acquiring a thorough experimental knowledge of some art or vocation which would render its possessor self-supporting and, consequently, independent.

If the tide of public opinion favoring such a course would but set in, many a one would be spared untold suffering and misery in after life. Let the rich set the example in this matter. They can afford to do whatever pleases them, and, therefore, have it in their power to mould public opinion. Be not afraid, girls, that you will find your self-imposed task irksome. Remember that occupation is necessary to happiness, and that there is no reason why you should not dream while you work. The cry will be raised that there is danger that such a plan as the one advocated here will tend to give girls a distaste for the quiet retirement of home, but there is little cause for fear. Not one girl in twenty will voluntarily choose a business life in preference to domestic happiness. Indeed, it is absolutely certain that happy marriages would be promoted by this very independence among women. Not being at leisure to nurse every passing fancy, girls would elect to wait patiently until the light of true love came into their lives.

C Andreas, May 1885

CHAPTER TWO

A New Profession For Women

The stranger in New York who may chance to visit the east side of the city in the neighborhood of 26th Street will have his attention called to a long, grayish, four-story prison-like structure, with a wing, situated in a block which extends to the East River, and enclosed by a high, forbidding stone wall. This is Bellevue Hospital, the chief free public institution of the kind in New York. For many years it has been famous for the high medical and surgical skill of which it is the theater, its faculty embracing many leading members of the profession in the city. For many years to come it is likely to be popularly associated with another high development of the curative arts, the results of the founding, in 1873, of the Bellevue Training School for Nurses, and of a new profession for women in America.

Not long ago, a lady living in the suburbs of one of our eastern cities, whose daughter was ill with fever, was urged by her physician to employ a professional nurse. She was loath to do this, but, as the malady increased in virulence, she finally yielded. The following morning the servant announced 'the nurse'.

To the mother's imagination, overwrought as it was by lack of rest and by unremitting watching, the words called up the most disagreeable anticipations of a careless and disorderly person, and perhaps even a dark reminiscence of Sairey Gamp scolding trembling invalids, removing their pillows, or drinking copiously from black bottles, while grim-visaged Betsey Prig looked on with unconcern.

With these pictures of the professional nurse before her, she descended to the hall. There, to her surprise, she found a young woman of intelligent face, neat apparel, and quiet demeanor.

'You are?'

'The nurse, madam.'

Saying which, the stranger exhibited a badge inscribed with the words Bellevue Hospital Training School for Nurses, and decorated with a stork, the emblem of watchfulness.

The physician now appearing, the nurse listened attentively to his instructions. Her movements, while preparing for duty, inspired with confidence both mother and patient. Her skillful hand prepared the food, her watchful eye anticipated every want. She was calm, patient, and sympathizing; but though eager to please and cheer the invalid, she did not stoop to simulate an affection she did not feel, nor to express hopes of recovery that could not be realized. The exaction, the impatience incident to illness, seemed but to incite her to renewed effort in behalf of her charge. She met every emergency with knowledge and unruffled spirit. To the physician, she proved an invaluable assistant, executing his orders intelligently, and recording accurately the various symptoms as they were developed. She watched the temperature of the room as closely as she did that of the patient, and while always polite and obliging, was never obsequious.

The mother had doubtless heard indirectly of the school of which her efficient nurse was a graduate, but she was, as many others are, unfamiliar with its work and aims.

To understand the almost revolutionary progress that, through the instrumentality of this school, has been made in the system of nursing the sick, let us look for a moment at the previous condition of this great hospital.

The present building was constructed about sixty years ago, by the poorhouse authorities; for thirty years it was an almshouse, and since then it has been used exclusively for hospital purposes. So unenlightened was the general view of the obligations of a city toward its sick and injured in those days, that for years the only nursing was done by convicts of the Female Penitentiary.

The profanity, drunkenness, theft, and profligacy of these attendants were soon too scandalous to be ignored, and in 1848 this system was abolished, and hired nurses, selected from among poor women of reputable character and decent habits, were employed in all the wards. The advance from no nursing to poor nursing told sensibly on the death-rate, which, however, owing to poor hospital supplies, bad ventilation and beds, defects of heating and cleanliness, and the general indifference to the welfare of the patients, still continued large; the best medical skill was useless against incompetence and neglect.

So matters continued until the year 1872, when the attention of the Local Visiting Committee of the New York State Charities Aid Association was called to Bellevue. This committee was composed of sixty members, chiefly ladies of high social position and intelligence, two visitors being assigned to each ward. Their duties were to visit the hospital weekly, and to report its actual condition to the Association.

They found in the building nine hundred patients, most of them in want, many in positive distress. The men's wards were so crowded that three patients would have to sleep on two beds and five on three. Others were forced to sleep on the floor without blankets or pillows, as there was no supply of extra clothing, except what could be obtained from the stock belonging to deceased patients. A few of the hired nurses were still there, and they seemed to have learned nothing by experience, save indifference to suffering.

There were no night nurses, and only three night watchmen for six hundred patients. They sometimes drugged the patients with morphine to keep them quiet, and drank the stimulants that had been prescribed.

In the kitchen, it was ascertained that tea and soup were frequently made in the same boiler; the coffee was nauseous, and the beef dry and hard. Special diet existed only in name, and even if ordered and provided, it had little chance of reaching the patients or even the nurses, being confiscated on the way up from the kitchen by the workhouse women, who had been committed for drunkenness or disorderly conduct, and had been transferred to Bellevue as helpers.

Judging from these inspections, the committee became convinced that no improvement could be hoped for in the management of the hospital until a complete reform of the nursing should be effected; and, inspired by the example and success of similar work in England by Florence Nightingale, the founder of the modern system of nursing, they set themselves to this task with resolution, tact, and intelligence.

At first they met with little encouragement from the medical profession, but now their staunchest supporters are found within it. One distinguished physician said,

'I do not believe in the success of a training-school for nurses at Bellevue. The patients are of a class so difficult to deal with, and the service is so laborious, that the conscientious, intelligent women you are looking for will lose heart and hope long before the two years of training are over.' [1] A clergyman well acquainted with the hospital echoed this opinion, and thought it was not a proper place for ladies to visit. One or two physicians thought the lives of such people not worth saving. Other grades of opposition or indifference presented themselves: political, social and professional.

The experiment was a new one, and the theory on which it was undertaken ran counter to the traditions of those employed in the hospital. Before such obstacles, stout hearts might well have hesitated, but the courageous and intelligent managers were only thereby the more firmly convinced of the necessity of patient and persistent effort.

---

[1] Exceptions to the general attitude were found in the cordial cooperation of the late Dr. James R. Wood, Dr. Austin Flint, and Dr. Stephen Smith, who were fast friends of the enterprise from the start, and have been of the greatest aid as advisers to the Board of Management.

The first step was to learn how to organize the school in the best way, and for this end, Dr. W. Gill Wylie, of New York, volunteered to go to Europe at his own expense, to study the foreign systems. Upon his return he brought a cordial letter from Miss Nightingale, in which she set forth the principles upon which the management of the school has been based. Chief of these is the entire subordination of the nursing corps to the medical staff, the nurses being under the discipline of a superintendent, or matron, whose duty it is to see that the work is performed to the satisfaction of the physicians. To her report the head-nurses, who have a surveillance of both the day and night nurses.

The position assigned to the matron, by which she is made solely responsible for the efficiency of the nursing corps, is one of the most important features. The tact and judgment displayed by the training-school managers in the practical application of these sensible ideas of the function of nursing, have saved a vast amount of friction, and won for the school the friendship of many physicians who were naturally prejudiced against it, and might easily have been forced into opposition by any encroachment upon their rights.

The boundaries of the nurses duties having been laid down with circumspection, voluntary subscriptions were called for and made to the amount of $23,000, and a house was rented near the hospital, in which the nurses should lodge and board.

To find a person capable of taking charge of such an institution proved a difficult task. Miss Bowden, otherwise known as Sister Helen, of All Saints, then of Baltimore, but formerly of the well-known school at University College, London, was finally selected.

Equal difficulty was experienced in procuring assistants for her. Advertisements were inserted in the journals, and physicians were applied to; but such was the scarcity of educated nurses in this country at that time, that, after a search of many months, and after the most liberal offers, only four were found who were in any wise capable, one of whom proved inefficient.

Later on, Sister Helen, compelled to return to England, was succeeded by Miss Perkins, of Norwich, Connecticut, under whose management the school has continued to increase in numbers and usefulness. At first but six pupils were obtained. The scheme adopted that developed by Miss Nightingale demanded in the applicant a combination of requisites the mere enumeration of which appalled many who had been encouraged to seek admission to the school.

These are: Good education, strong constitution, freedom from physical defects, including those of sight and hearing, and unexceptionable references. The course of training consists in dressing wounds, applying fomentations, bathing and care of helpless patients, making beds, and managing positions. Then follow the preparation and application of bandages, making rollers and linings of splints. The nurse must also learn how to prepare, cook, and serve delicacies for the invalid.

Instruction is given in the best practical methods of supplying fresh air, and of warming and ventilating the sick-room. In order to remain through the two years course and obtain a diploma, still more is required, viz.: Exemplary deportment, patience, industry, and obedience.

The first year's experience was far from satisfactory. Among seventy-three applicants, hailing from the various States, only twenty-nine were found that gave promise of ability to fulfill the conditions. Of these, ten were dismissed for various causes before the expiration of the first nine months.

To serve medicine to the patients in the wards of a great public hospital smacks not a little of novelty and of romance, and goes far, at first, to compensate for a hospital's unpleasant surroundings and its odour of disinfectants; but a short period of wound-dressing and night-watching is sufficient to dispel such illusions.

Every year, young women whose abilities warranted their admittance at the commencement of the course have been permitted to depart before its completion, owing to an evident distaste on their part for the duties imposed upon them.

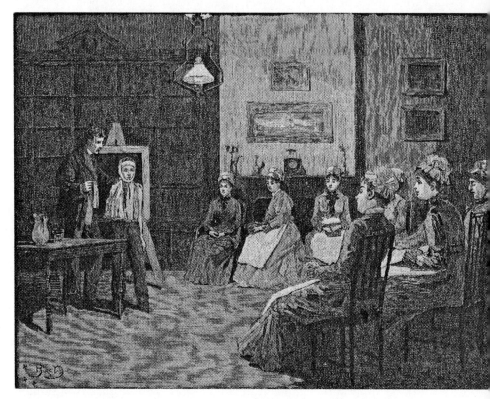

A demonstration in Bandaging at Bellevue

But the managers, though surprised at the result of their first efforts, were not discouraged. As time went by, the number of applicants increased, and, though the high standard first established was not departed from, the proportion of those capable of fulfilling the requirements multiplied. Some applicants, who did not seem especially adapted to the work, proved most efficient, and on this topic the managers say that, after their long experience, they have found that the fitness of an applicant can be determined only by absolute trial.

The nurses at the Bellevue school may be divided into two classes: those who study the art of nursing with a view to gaining a livelihood or supporting their families, and those who look forward to a life of usefulness among the poor sick. All are lodged and boarded free of charge during the two years course, and are paid a small sum monthly, while in the school, to defray their actual necessary expenses, and, in order to avoid all distinction between rich and poor, every nurse is expected to receive this pay.

The Nurses Home, the Headquarters of the school, is No.426 East 26th Street, a large and handsome building, erected for the purpose and given to the school by Mrs. W. H. Osborn. From the outside of this building, the tastefully arranged curtains and polished panes of its several chambers present a striking contrast to the sombre, frowning walls of the great charity hospital opposite.

Besides studying from text-books, and attending a systematic course of lectures, the pupils are occupied by the care of the patients in the hospital, and in the general management of the wards. The nurses are taught how to make accurate observations and reports of symptoms for the physicians use, such as state of pulse, temperature, appetite, intelligence, delirium or stupor, breathing, sleep, condition of wounds, effect of diet, medicine, or stimulant. This instruction is given by the visiting and resident physicians and surgeons of Bellevue, at the bedside of the patients, and by the super-intendent and head-nurse.

At first, only the female wards were supplied; but, as illness makes no distinction of sex, it was found impossible to complete the nurse's education without practice among sick men, and early in the career of the institution, some of the male wards were included, until now 14 wards of from 6 to 20 beds each are under the supervision of the new system. There is no reason, except the want of money, why this system should not be extended to the entire hospital.

Look in at the male surgical ward. These young women in white caps and aprons and blue-and-white striped seersucker dresses seem to have had something of the training of the soldier added to that of the nurse. There is little talking and no laughing. When they do speak, it is in subdued tones. Each seems to understand her duties. One of the house physicians enters, and, beckoning to a nurse, gives her directions regarding a particular patient recently visited. She listens attentively, makes no reply, and turns at once to obey.

A soldier, pausing in his rounds, presenting arms to his superior officer and listening respectfully for orders, would not have exhibited a more perfect discipline. On either hand, the patients lie on their cots, in the various stages of relapse or recovery. As a rule, these are hard-featured, ill-favored men. Some are only waiting here until the healing of their wounds to be tried for felonious assault, housebreaking, or murder. One is a barkeeper, brought in the previous night in an ambulance, after a melee in which he was shot through the chest. His face wears a puzzled expression as the nurse quietly and skillfully dresses the wound; such kind attention is a revelation to him.

In the next cot, is a man who has been run over, while intoxicated, by a truck. His injuries are serious, and require the almost undivided attention of a skilled nurse; if she had not been at hand, the surgeon would be obliged to amputate the leg that now swings easily upon the strap-support.

On the opposite side of the ward, stretched upon a cot near the door, is a workman who has been injured by falling from a scaffold. He has a care-worn, anxious expression that proceeds not from physical, but mental troubles. He has just told the nurse that his wife is very ill, and that there is no one to look after her and the children. He does not know, but will soon learn, that another young woman with even more experience than the one sitting near him, is already on her way to his wife, the number of his house having been ascertained from the hospital entry-book on the ground floor.

In another division of this ward are gathered the most complicated cases. The labors of the nurse must here be unremitting; yet little medicine is required. Some of these poor fellows who lie in rows are, doubtless, beyond the influence of that, but the world is still sweet to them, and the spark of life that fitfully lights up their wan, colorless faces may, if carefully tended, still be kept aglow.

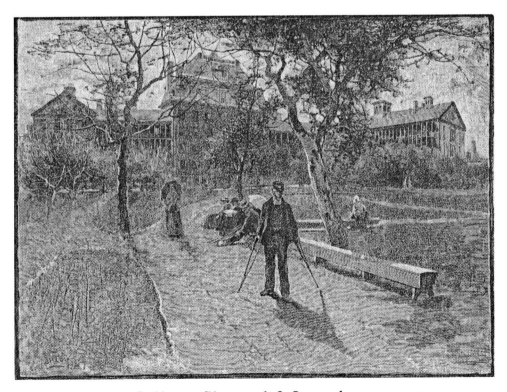

Bellevue Hospital & Grounds

One patient is undergoing an operation, though not a dangerous one. The nurse stands by, supporting his head and shoulders. Ether is not required, but the man has been already broken down with his malady; his face twitches with pain, his hands open and shut convulsively, and a groan escapes him, deep, prolonged, and expressive not only of present pain, but of the weary months of suffering that he has experienced. Now the surgeon's work is done, and the poor fellow, before sinking back again upon his pillow, murmurs a stuttering apology to the nurse for having shown what he takes to be weakness while under the lancet.

In the female wards, the work of the trained nurses is employed to better purpose probably than elsewhere within the walls of the institution. The old and the young hobble about on crutches, or lie on their cots with blanched, careworn faces, and deep-sunken eyes. A kindly faced nurse is feeding an old woman from a bowl. Whatever it contains, it causes a smile to light up what before had been sullen and frigid features. Another is carefully bandaging a wounded arm, striving, meanwhile, to argue away from the sufferer the spectre that haunts her. The most uninviting and wretched tenement-houses do not reveal a class more in need of help and sympathy than the patients in the female wards of Bellevue.

The bell of an ambulance which has just arrived strikes three startling strokes, the signal for the medical division. A few minutes pass, and two men bring in a stretcher, on which rests the form of a woman clad in genteel but much-worn apparel. Two nurses lift the motionless form upon a bed, and examine the card made out for each patient upon her arrival. It is super-scribed 'No Friends', and a careful examination of the small leather bag tightly clasped in her hand fails to furnish additional intelligence.

She was found lying insensible upon the pavement, and, though she regained consciousness for a few minutes previous to the arrival of the ambulance, she stubbornly refused to answer questions, to give her name, or tell what ailed her. But the nurses soon discovered this trouble.

The woman was starving: she had been starving herself purposely. She had had some misfortune, of which she refused to speak. Her first words upon recovering consciousness were of regret that she had not been permitted to die. Later on, however, she was encouraged to partake of nourishing food. With this and good nursing, her spirits to a certain extent revived, until, upon her departure, she had, to all appearance, ceased to reflect upon that which had caused her distress.

Upon the completion of their labors in the Training-School, and after passing a satisfactory examination, the nurses, furnished with diplomas, signed by the managers and the examining board of the hospital, begin their several careers. Some are called to superintend state and city hospitals, a continually increasing number seek private practice, or rather are sought by it, while not a few, as has already been said, devote themselves to the sick among the poor.

The value of the service performed by these noble women cannot be adequately estimated without visiting the tenement-house district wherein it is performed. They lodge in a house provided for the purpose by the Woman's Branch of the City Missions, by which they are supported, and are to New York what the District Nurses are to London.

From early morning until evening, they endure fatigue, heat, cold, and storm, in their efforts to relieve the distressed. Neither the gruff responses, nor the ingratitude of those for whom they toil, have, in a single known instance, forced them to cease their work. An equally zealous person, without the advantages of a nurses training, would fail signally where she would succeed.

For the mere attendance on the invalid is not the whole of the service performed by the visiting nurse. She sweeps and cleans the rooms, cooks the food, does the washing, if necessary, goes upon errands - in short, takes the place of the mother, if she be ill. All this has been learned at the training-school. Neither illness nor death itself can appall her: she has served a long novitiate in nursing the one, and the other has long since lost its terrors.

Here is the substance of an account given by one of these charitable women, of a typical days work.

'I heard that a young man was dying of consumption in a tenement-house on the eastside. After searching for some time, I found the house, squeezed in between two larger and equally dilapidated structures, in the rear of those facing the street. It had no door, and, like such houses generally, was so dark, even in broad daylight, that I had to grope my way to the upper chambers by aid of the stair rail. A woman in the yard told me that the man I wished to see lodged, she thought, on the top floor.

'Upon my arrival, I knocked for some time at the doors of the front chambers, but no one answered. Then I tried the back hall-room.

'Who's there?' a man's voice roughly demanded.

'I want to speak with you,' I answered.

'Well, who are you?'

'I said that I would explain my business, if he would open the door, and, after a few moments, it was opened just a few inches. The face of a little, weazened old man appeared.

'What do you want?' he demanded, scowlingly.

'I heard there was an invalid here, and I want to try and do something for him.'

'Well, he doesn't want anything.'

But, I persisted,

'Can't I see him for a moment?'

'No, you can't.'

'He would have slammed the door in my face, but I had caught sight of the poor fellow, his son, who was crouched in one corner.

I beckoned to him, and he unwillingly came toward the door in time to prevent its being closed.

'Don't you like beef-tea?' I asked.

'No, I don't,' he returned.

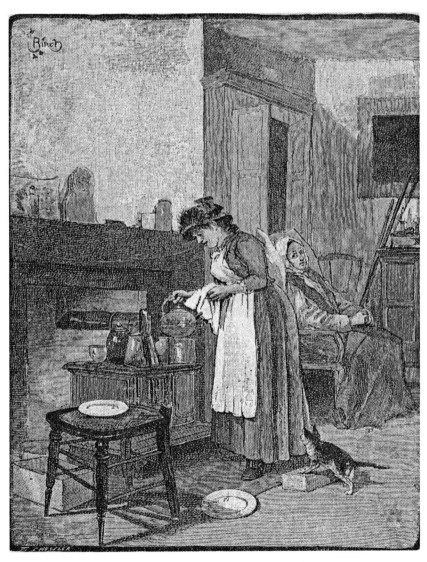

Tenement-House Work

'But I have some here that you will like. I'm sure it's different from what you've seen. Let me make some for you. You needn't take it, if you don't like it.'

'I don't know,' he said. 'I might.'

'And, despite the scowls of the father, who was opposed to my entrance, I sat down by the stove, gathered some pieces of wood from a pile in the corner, and made a fire warm enough to heat the beef-tea. The young man was in the last stages of consumption, and said he had not eaten anything for sometime, though I saw some bits of dry bread and pork upon an adjoining shelf. He had no sooner tasted the tea I made for him than he smacked his lips with evident surprise and pleasure, and declared it very good. It seemed to warm him up mentally as well as physically, seeing which, I plied him with questions regarding his illness and means of support, questions which, notwithstanding the evident displeasure of his father, he answered courteously and intelligently.

'Before my departure I put the room in order, and brought to the invalid and his father sufficient good food for a few days, and showed them how to prepare it.

'My next visit was to a little boy who had been run over while playing in the street. He was dead when I reached him, and his mother, worn out alike by mental and physical exhaustion, for she had not slept at all, and had eaten but little for several days, was lying moaning upon a bed. Another child lay in an adjoining room, quite ill with malarial fever.

'This is so prevalent among tenement-house children in warm weather, that we usually carry with us something to relieve them. So I did what I could for her, and then began to arrange the rooms and prepare the dinner. The mother appeared indifferent to what was taking place; but the father, a truck-driver by profession, who sat silent at the window, seemed much pleased with my efforts.

'The rooms were close and the atmosphere was permeated with bad air coming from the lower halls. The back windows looked into those of ill-kept, tumbledown structures across a court, the odours of which were alike offensive.

'The family clothes were suspended upon some of the ropes that formed a sort of cob-web between the adjoining buildings. They had remained hanging there for nearly a week, and after serving the dinner, I set about taking them in. This was no easy matter. While tugging upon the lines, they caught upon those belonging to the inmates of the other houses, and clogged up the pulley, and, before I had completed my labors, I had been roundly scolded for my awkwardness by the stout, red-faced occupants of the windows in the quadrangle.

'The cart-man had been compelled to remain home and neglect his work for several days, in order to assist his wife. His money was almost gone in consequence, at a time, too, when an unusual outlay was necessary. So I returned early the following day, and remained until the affairs of the household were again in smooth-running order.

'The most unsatisfactory visits we make are to those addicted to the use of intoxicating liquor. It was upon one of these I next called. In a little, dingy apartment in the wing of an old house which seemed to lean for support upon its neighbor, equally unsteady, I found a woman whose children I had nursed for weeks at a time. I had before seen her when under the influence of liquor, but now she seemed to be almost crazed with it.

The children, ragged and dirty, were lying upon the floor, and, when I offered to look after them during her absence - for she was putting on her bonnet - she almost flew at me, with taunts that I had abandoned her when she was starving. As a matter of fact, I had been with her upon the previous day.'

Such is the work, such the experience of those of the training-school graduates who elect to exchange the comforts (often the luxuries) of home, and the society of friends, for the exposures and dangers incident to a life among the poor sick.

When the managers of the training-school announced, some years since, that they would send nurses to private families in cases of illness, the applications were so few that they were led to fear that this branch of the school would be unsupported, and that the nurses would find themselves deceived regarding their future prospects. But the value of the trained nurse, little known at that time in America, soon began to be recognized, and the demand for such services increased, until, at the present time, there is a greater call for nurses than can be supplied. Many who formerly refused to consider a suggestion to call in a nurse, now eagerly apply for them; and surgeons, in certain instances, have refused to perform operations without the subsequent assistance of a trained nurse.

Before going to a private house, the nurse is carefully instructed by the superintendent. She must not leave it without communicating with her, nor return from her duties without a certificate of conduct and efficiency from the family of the patient or the physician attending. She is expected and urged to bear in mind the importance of the situation, and to show, at all times, self-denial and forbearance. She must take upon herself the entire charge of the sick-room.

Above all, she is charged to hold sacred any knowledge of its private affairs which she may acquire through her temporary connection with the household. She receives a stipulated sum for her services, but this will not always compensate her for the annoyances with which the position is occasionally beset.

In addition to this field in New York City and vicinity, there is an increasing demand throughout the country for experienced nurses to take charge of hospitals and schools.

Graduates of the Bellevue school have been called to be superintendents of the nursing departments of the following institutions:

Massachusetts General Hospital; Boston City Hospital; New Haven City Hospital; New York Hospital; Mt. Sinai Hospital, New York City; Brooklyn City Hospital; Cook County Hospital, Chicago; St. Luke's Hospital, Denver; Charity Hospital, New Orleans, and the Minneapolis (Minn.) Hospital; others are matrons of Roosevelt Hospital, New York City; Charleston (S. C.) Hospital; Lawrence (Mass.) Hospital, and the Seaman's Hospital, Savannah, Ga.

Thus has the great work set afoot by a few noble women of New York developed, little by little, amid difficulties of which it would he useless to complain, since all have been surmounted. The results have amply justified their conviction that a demand for efficient nurses would speedily follow their supply, and that American women could be found willing to nurse the pauper sick, provided they were at the same time assured of a competence.

That the profession of trained nurse will rise in estimation as the value of her services becomes better known, there is little doubt. Other occupations than hers have successfully met and overcome prejudice. Less than two centuries ago, the English clergy were entertained in the servant's hall, were sent upon errands, and were expected to marry my lady's waiting-maid. It was later yet when the surgeon was separated from the barber, as that by no means ancient pile, the Barber-Surgeons hall, still standing in London may remind us.

Against any such lingering prejudice, the moral and professional character of the school will prove an ample defence. Founded in the belief that the value of a nurse is in proportion to her intelligence, capacity, and refinement, it has proved an important step forward in our civilization, and its standard is not likely to be lowered in order to make a show of graduates.

During the nine years of its existence, one hundred and forty-nine pupils have received diplomas, seventy-eight of whom are now practicing in New York City. Perhaps twice as many capable women have been turned away because the school cannot he further enlarged until the financial support of the enterprise is more considerable than at present.

In conclusion it must he said that, while Miss Nightingale's theories are the basis of the Training-School, its managers have found it necessary to depart from the English system in some important particulars. For instance, Miss Nightingale regards it as indispensable that the superintendent and the nurses should live within the hospital.

Our experience is the reverse of this, say the committee. American women, being of a sensitive, nervous organization, are at first depressed by the painful aspects of hospital life, and when they become interested in the work they take it greatly to heart. Hence it is of importance to have a cheerful, comfortable home where they can each day throw off the cares of their profession. To the restfulness of the Home is attributed the exceptional health of the nurses, among whom but one death and very few dangerous illnesses have occurred since the opening of the school, almost ten years ago.

Another necessity in an American training-school is the abolition of caste. In England the ward sister (who has received thorough training) is expected to be a lady, superior in social position and intelligence to the nurses, who are drawn from the class of domestic servants.

At Bellevue, the preliminary examination, and the high standard subsequently exacted, exclude, and are meant to exclude them. But among those who enter there is no distinction. All submit to the same discipline and perform the same duties, none of which, being connected with the sick, is considered menial.

Note: The introduction of trained nurses into county poorhouses is a natural sequence of their successful introduction into this hospital department of a city almshouse. In many poorhouses but little or no care is taken of the sick, one of the least disabled paupers usually being put in charge of those more seriously ill. Not in vain has the State Charities Aid Association called public attention to this state of things. The old barbarisms are passing away and a new era is at hand. New York City wears the proud laurel of having first introduced trained nursing into a city almshouse, as Rensselaer County (Troy) leads the van of its introduction into a county poorhouse. The authorities of this poorhouse have recently engaged a graduate of the Bellevue School to take charge of the nursing department, and it is hoped that other counties of the State of New York may follow this humane example.

Franklin D North, November 1882

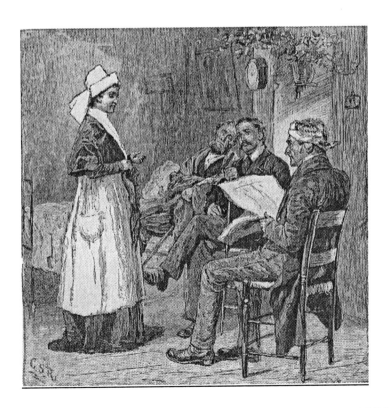

Convalescents, Homeopathic Hospital, Brooklyn, 1878

CHAPTER THREE
The Connecticut Training School for Nurses

A new idea usually finds simultaneous development in several directions, and it is rare that one person alone is the discoverer. The common parent of American hospital schools is the Nightingale Memorial of St. Thomas's Hospital, London; but the plan for their organization here was common to several communities.

For example, the New Haven School was developed, a small endowment raised, and the charter obtained, simultaneously with the Bellevue Hospital School -though chance prevented the reception of pupils in New Haven until six months later.

A school of the size of the New Haven School, adapted to the wants of a comparatively small, hospital, stands in relation to similar organizations in large charity hospitals as the private select school does to the large public ones in the common-school system.

In a hospital of only one hundred and sixty beds, there is no great mass of sick to care for; nurses have time to study the accomplishments of their profession, and lady visitors and managers are able to give personal attention and supervision to the classes. That the results are favorable is shown in the New Haven School by the number, in proportion to the graduate, who have been called to fill positions of trust in other hospitals, nearly one-fourth having been given the supervision of nursing in hospitals, in New Haven, New York City, Brooklyn, Pittsfield (Massachusetts), Boston, and the States of New Jersey, Indiana, Ohio, Vermont, and Virginia.

The growth of the school in public favor is shown by the constantly increasing demand for nurses for private families, two-thirds in excess of the provision, and also by the applications for admissions, which at the present moment are greatly in excess of the vacancies. Another proof of the favor with which the enterprise is regarded is found in the liberal way in which money has lately been contributed to build in 'the hospital enclosure a nurses' home, now finished and occupied, having accommodations for thirty,- a handsome, ample three-story brick building, with cheerful parlors, single bedrooms, bathrooms, piazzas, etc., well-warmed, ventilated, and lighted, which -it may be useful to those engaged in similar undertakings to know - has been substantially and satisfactorily completed at an outside cost of $15,500.

It might be supposed that the New Haven School, comparatively small as it is, would have a local reputation only; it is noticeable, however, that young women all over the country are increasingly interested in the new profession open to them, and anxious to collect information concerning all the schools. Thus far the following places have been represented in the New Haven School by accepted pupils: Connecticut, Vermont, Maine, New Hampshire, Massachusetts, Rhode Island, New York, New Jersey, Michigan, Pennsylvania, Maryland, Georgia, Illinois, Wisconsin, Washington, Canada, Nova Scotia, and Australia.

Trained nurses have been sent on application to all the New England States, New York, Florida, and Virginia, - and on graduation have scattered to all quarters, from Canada to California.

For the benefit of those who may be desirous of connecting a nursing school with smaller hospitals than those found in our large cities, it may be useful to give the points of difference between the New Haven organization and similar undertakings in New York and Boston.

The New Haven School is in charge of a president, vice-presidents, general treasurer, and auditors, and a committee of twenty-one ladies and gentlemen, five being physicians, two of whom are connected with the hospital staff; this makes a connecting link between the ladies' committee and medical and other male boards of hospital management. The gentleman who is the general treasurer pays out to the sub-treasurer, who is a lady, the funds necessary for the current expense of the school, which she accounts for, making weekly payments to the nurses. The secretary, another member of the ladies' committee, conducts all the correspondence with applicants, accepts them if they answer the requirements, and notifies the lady superintendent when to expect new arrivals.

The assumption by the ladies' committee of all these duties relieves the superintendent of much outside responsibility and gives her time for her legitimate duties as instructor of the pupils in the wards. That the pupils may be under the best teaching it is required that the superintendent of nursing and her assistant shall themselves be ladies of thorough hospital training, knowing the theory and practice of skillful nursing, and able to recognize at once bungling work on the part of the pupils and to set them right.

In a small hospital it is unnecessary that ward head-nurses should be employed, as in large institutions, at an increased expense. Here the senior nurse in each ward is in that position, at the ordinary payment. Each pupil, coming in turn to be senior nurse, gains greatly in self-possession and quick perception -faculties which are required in this responsible position.

The hospital contributes nothing towards the payment of the nurses; that is attended to by the society. The table for the school is, however, provided by the hospital; and the officers; relieved from the daily cares of housekeeping, give their whole time to the supervision of the nursing. Differing again from other schools, the course of instruction here is shortened to nineteen months, thirteen spent in hospital and six at private nursing; this private nursing is required of all pupils.

In this way, the school receives additions to its funds in payments from families, and the committee know from actual trial and report whether the nurse is entitled to her diploma. The exigencies of very large hospitals make it necessary often to decline to send nurses to private families. The New

Haven School re quires that all should serve in this way for six months, their places in the hospital being taken by new pupils.

In all these ways - in the absence of increased payments toward head-nurses, and of housekeeping cares, and in the requirement of nursing in private families –the school finds an advantage over other systems.

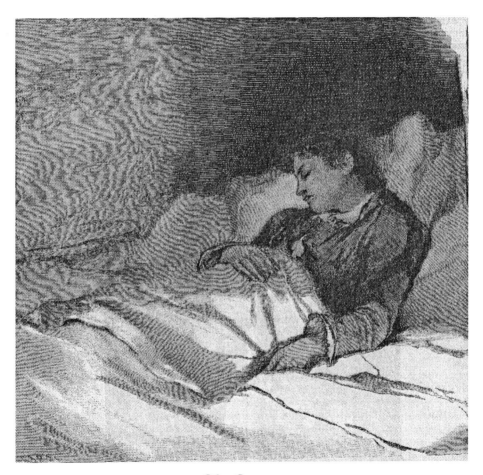

The Patient

One other difference is in the form of graduation papers. Each graduate receives with her diploma a printed statement of her standing in the school during her course of study, and the seal of the school is not affixed to the diploma until one year after graduation. At this time, the self-reliance of the nurse having been tested for this additional twelve months, a certain number of testimonials from physicians are required to be returned with the diploma for final action, and if a majority of the committee so decide the seal is affixed.

The course of instruction consists of careful teaching in the ward by the lady superintendent; recitations held daily from text-books, lectures, autopsies, attendance at surgical operations, and three weeks or more spent in the diet kitchen. Quarterly examinations are held and a prize is given for the best recitation. Examinations for diplomas are conducted by one of the physicians of the committee.

The school has published a hand-book of nursing, which is in use in the hospital schools of New York, Brooklyn, Chicago, Washington, and Orange, and in one of the large English hospital schools. It may be an encouragement to other schools in their beginning to see at the close of ten years how far a little candle throws its beams.

It is important to those about organizing a nursing school to lay special stress upon the need of strong health in their pupils. Only about one-third of all the accepted pupils of the New Haven School have finished their hospital course; and the cause of failure in a large majority of cases has been ill health. The work makes a drain upon the system mentally and physically, and it often happens that physicians who do not understand the wearing nature of hospital life will certify to the physical fitness of a young woman who in six months' time breaks down entirely, and the result is loss of health to her and loss of time and money to the school. Some applicants who bring clean bills of health from home are pronounced by our own physician unequal to the strain.

One other difference between this school and others is in the requirement that at the close of a year's hospital life the pupils shall take a month's vacation, to be spent away from the hospital. This is considered necessary, in order that pupils may go in a good physical condition to their nursing in private families.

The 'sources of financial support' are a small endowment and payments made by families for the services of nurses.

There is no hospital too small to furnish useful training to at least three or four pupil nurses, and all over the country there is a demand for skilled services in illness.

The New Haven School began in a very small way a few years ago, with six pupils, and has now over forty under its control, with a graduate list of more than one hundred. What is a far better test of success, however, than mere numbers, is the wide reputation it has secured for faithful training; and this reputation can be obtained by even the smallest cottage hospital.

October 1885

CHAPTER FOUR

The Training of a Nurse

Within the memory of most of us, nearly every family boasted some member who was said to be a born nurse, who came to the fore in times of sickness, and whose labor of love was sometimes shared by a paid outsider, usually a motherly body supposed to have a great deal of experience. But that time is past, and now no one who can afford a trained nurse thinks of taking a patient through an illness without one, any more than a captain willingly takes his ship through a dangerous channel without a pilot.

This means that a new trade or profession has been created for women, and it may be told once more that they owe it to one of the noblest women of her time.

At the close of the Crimean War, the passionate gratitude of the English people to Florence Nightingale found expression in a great public meeting, at which fifty thousand pounds was subscribed as a testimonial to her. She refused, however, to take it for herself, and at her request it was devoted to a foundation which was quaintly termed 'An Institution for the Training, Sustenance, and Protection of Nurses and Hospital Attendants', in connection with St. Thomas's Hospital, London; and thus the first English training school for nurses was started in June, 1860.

Accounts of this great reform, which spread in England from year to year, reached this country more or less vaguely, but were without result until, in 1872, the men and women belonging to that branch of the State Charities Aid Association which visited the sick in Bellevue Hospital felt that they could not do any good or lasting work until the existing system, or want of system, should be entirely changed. The nurses were too few in number, nearly all illiterate, some immoral, and others intemperate, and had sought their places simply as a means of livelihood, and not because they had any aptitude for, or knowledge of, their profession.

36

The members of the Bellevue Association therefore applied to the Commissioners of Charities and Correction for permission to establish a school for nurses at Bellevue Hospital, pledging themselves to pay the additional salaries and all other expenses of a better class of women and to put two more nurses in each ward.

The consent of the Medical Board of the hospital, to whom the Commissioners referred this appeal, having finally been given to what many physicians considered a doubtful experiment, the Bellevue Training School for Nurses was started on May 1, 1873, with a superintendent and five nurses, having five wards under their care.

In 1890, the school has 62 pupils and has graduated 345, while as a direct out-growth of that modest beginning there are three other great schools in New York alone. These are the New York City, which has 64 pupils and has graduated 263; the New York Hospital, with 48 pupils and 192 graduates; and Mount Sinai, with 50 pupils and 111 graduates. There are also smaller schools in the city, but, great or small, Bellevue must always be honored as the pioneer.

Her graduates are at the head of most of the important schools and hospitals in the country, and have even gone so far afield as England, Italy, and China.

The next school to be established was the New York City, which was started by the Commissioners of Charities and Correction in 1877, and is entirely supported by the City. Until last year it was known as the Charity Hospital School, because it began there, but as it grew its work spread until the old name was misleading and had to be changed.

It is now the largest and in some respects the most important of all the schools, as it nurses five different hospitals: Charity and Maternity on Blackwell's Island, the Infants Hospital on Randall's Island, Gouverneur at Gouverneur Slip, and Harlem; at the foot of East 120th Street, the two last being accident or emergency hospitals, while at Charity the cases are largely chronic.

Besides the pupils of the school, there are 32 permanent trained nurses at Charity and Randall's Island, making nearly a hundred in all, for whom the superintendent is directly responsible, and over whom she has full authority. The other schools in the city are supported from the funds of the hospitals which they nurse.

I have said that nursing is a trade or profession, for it is really both being a trade, in that it exacts manual skill and dexterity, and a profession because it requires mental ability, judgment, and progressive knowledge. The hospital is therefore at once a workshop and a college, with this essential difference, however, that its scholars exist because it has need of them, not they of it.

So much talk has been made about nursing as a noble vocation that it is easy to lose sight of the fact that hospital training schools are run first of all because hospital patients must be taken care of. When Florence Nightingale led her little band of workers out of England it was not in order that women should have a new vocation, but because men were dying like flies in the hospitals at Scutari, and the women who started the Bellevue School did so because they found the hospital could be well nursed in no other way.

In most of the schools, the nurses receive each $10 a month during the first year of their service, and $15 the second, and at the present time there is some discussion as to whether they should be paid at all, or should give their time in return for their professional training, as the house physicians do.

This seems reasonable enough to an outsider, but in the first place much of a nurses work is of a routine kind, repeated far oftener than is necessary for her education, and such as a doctor is rarely called upon to do, and in the second, the most desirable pupils are those who could be self-supporting outside the schools, and will not be a burden on their families while in them.

In this country, there is a large class of conscientious and industrious women whose education and early associations lead them to look for some higher and more thoughtful labor than household service or work in shops, who have received the good education of our common schools, and who are dependent on their own exertions for support. These women can be trained to make the best possible nurses, and it is the unanimous opinion of the superintendents of the large schools that it would be false economy to seek to deprive such pupils of the small salary which now keeps them independent during two years of very hard work.

We will suppose that a woman of this kind has decided to go into one of the large schools, and has applied to the superintendent for information. She receives in return a circular giving the rules, requirements, and course of study, and in due time finds herself with other candidates waiting for examination in the superintendent's office. When her turn comes, and if her credentials are satisfactory, the superintendent usually talks to her a little while in order to find out what grade of nurse she is likely to make; for candidates are admitted only on their own merits, and where there are more applicants than vacancies it is important to secure the best.

A short examination in spelling, dictation, and simple arithmetic follows, and also in reading aloud, but this is often passed over if the candidate is evidently too nervous to do herself justice.

Various experiments have been tried as to Examining Boards, but the best result is always gained by choosing a good superintendent, and then leaving her free to select her own nurses, without fear or favor, from those who present themselves, as she must train, discipline, and live with them for two years, and has therefore every reason to take only those who are likely to do her credit.

Apart from articles in professional journals, much that has been written about hospital life is apt to strike one familiar with it as somewhat vague and sentimental, and there may therefore be some interest in the following sketches, by pupils now in the New York City Training School. The first gives a general outline of the work.

'We each begin our duty in the hospital as probationers on a month's trial. That beginning is very new to most of us; quite unlike anything in our previous lives. Before entering the school, some of us may have imagined that we had a peculiar fitness for nursing, even if we did not consider ourselves born nurses. We may have made up our minds that we knew how to make a poultice, and to care for the sick by being kind to them and ventilating their rooms.

'We may possibly have read Miss Nightingales Notes and so are quite sure that we know something of nursing; but that the hospital training will give us a sort of standing, and therefore it will be a desirable thing to have. As we proceed with our training, we discover that we did not know how to make a poultice, nor how best to care for a sick person.

'Some of us, again, know nothing at all about nursing, but we are not required to know anything. A head nurse prefers to train the raw material, so to speak, in her own way.

'What is required is that the probationer be receptive, that she be intelligent and, above all, active; and in case she has any knowledge of nursing, or ideas, or opinions, if she is discriminating she will keep them to herself.

'We have no dreaming time; there is no place for sentiment, and very little for sympathy in the ordinary sense of the word. Were we to sympathize with all the woes that we see we should be used up, we should die.

'A probationer enters the ward for the first time, and is introduced to her head nurse. She is then probably set to do some simple piece of work, such as arranging a closet or folding clothes and the like. On the next day she will have her regular duties to learn. As the afternoon goes on she may find

40

herself looking at the clock watching for 5.30 P.M. to come so that she may go off duty, and she has, probably, a bad headache.

'There is a hospital atmosphere, produced by the smell of drags and other unavoidable odors, perceptible to a fresh nose; there are strange sights and sounds which, combined, give a sort of shock for the first day. The new nurse may not be able to sleep that night, and by the end of the week she may find herself crying in bed, with pain in her feet and legs. These little ailments she keeps to herself. She is anxious to give satisfaction, and she has to do unquestioningly all that she is directed to do. A head nurse is nearly always considerate, if necessary helping her through with her work and encouraging her.

'Time goes on and the probationer becomes a junior, a senior, and finally a head nurse, and as we proceed with our training, each day, if we will, we can learn something; we gain confidence in ourselves and others gain confidence in us.

'I suppose we are rather an ordinary class of young women. We never talk of ideals; we may not even think of them; perhaps we have not any. We are essentially matter of fact; we have to deal with human beings and with facts. Our two years service to most of us is a means to an end, and that a material one, viz.: the earning of money.

'Someone told us at our commencement that we had done well to have chosen a profession which would not go out of fashion and which could not be done by machinery. That is a good start anyway.

'I am speaking of us as a whole; in the school we are told we cease to be individuals. That does not mean that we become automatic, for, I suppose there is no calling for women which needs more personality, more individuality.

'Whatever may have been the rush, monotony, or otherwise of our day (and there are some days in which everything seems out of joint), when our time to be relieved comes, we go away from the hospital, and if we choose we need not give it another thought for the next twelve hours.

Out of the hospital we have not a care, unless it is for ourselves; we know how to appreciate our leisure; we are cheerful and apparently happy, and sometimes frivolous; in fact, we are quite sisterly, as behooves all good nurses to be.

Our training is divided into what we call services. We have so many months training in the different services. They are medical, surgical, maternity, gynecological, eye, skin and throat, and the care of infants. About six months of our time is spent on night duty, spread over the two years in periods of about six weeks duration. The large wards of Charity Hospital have each four nurses two juniors, one senior, and a head nurse. In the emergency hospitals, a nurse has usually the charge of a ward by herself, with a supervising nurse over all. There are also special cases, the patient having a room to himself, and a day and a night nurse appointed in charge. We each have our preferences and our dislikes, which are of no account as far as the distribution of the services is concerned; it makes us something to talk of, but we are under discipline; we go where we are sent.

'We begin our duties in a large ward of Charity Hospital. The probationer will have charge of one side of the ward, with the care of from ten to fifteen patients and all belonging to them. The head or senior nurse will go round with her and work in with her for the first time. She is shown how to make the beds, to change all soiled linen; how to remove a very sick patient from one bed to another; how to cover a patient and save her from fatigue while sitting up to have her bed made; the best way for her to get in and out of bed; to keep an eye on the beds that the patients are able to make themselves, and so on throughout the details of the morning's work.

'The latter part of the day is taken up with waiting on the patients and keeping her side in order all the time. The probation month is especially a time of learning something new; a good deal has to be got into that month; afterward things come more by degrees. Should the probationer be accepted, she becomes a junior nurse and has the same kind of work for about three months.

'She then goes on night duty; she is on the landing as we call it, that is, has charge of the two or three of the wards opening on to that landing. The junior nurse is feeling somewhat independent and consequential by this time. She does not have to act by herself; there is always an experienced nurse on the top floor to whom she can refer in case of emergency or otherwise.

'A nurse may never have been up all night in her life before, so the first night is rather exciting and anxious; she is very wide awake until about two or three o'clock in the morning when the effort to keep awake is really painful. A night nurse does not sleep, that goes without saying, and should she doze when all is quiet she has always one ear open. Imagine a rather young nurse peering around the large ward with the aid of an antiquated lantern. Shall I ever forget that lantern? It would throw all shadow and the least possible ray of light and anywhere but where it was wanted.

'Sometimes its miserable little light would go out and the wick have to be pricked up and relit, then it would spit and splutter as though it meant to burn well, but somehow it never would, and the gas burnt low on the landing. When I think of that lantern I can go all through my night duty over again. We have a helper to fetch and carry for us, and she can be very useful in many ways. She may be as good as a nurse or she may have a fancy for gossiping with her friends during the day and so prefer to sleep at night, and such a lady is rather a trial.

'The patients have a way of dying at night, in spite of the very best efforts of the nurse to keep them alive until morning. Some helpers never could go aside a dead body, but they don't mind fetching the things and standing outside of the screen. It requires considerable nerve on the part of the nurse to lay out a patient in the small hours of the morning; when the wards are silent and gloomy there is something uncanny about it; there is not much of the beauty of death in these cases, but we get used to it after a time.

'When we become more experienced, we have our emergency hospital night duty. We occasionally speak of this in rather strong language; we call it that awful night duty, that dreadful night duty. Here is where a nurse's mettle comes in. She has long hours, fourteen, and besides the care of the patients she has the real ward work to get done before eight o'clock in the morning.

'The patients in this hospital are very sick; there are no chronics, the nurse has critical cases to watch, and upon her devotion and judgment the life of the patient may depend. Here the doctors are hard worked both day and night, and the nurse, if she is considerate, is very reluctant to call the doctor, and so often has an anxious time. Some of the cases that come in during the night are truly heart-rending. The burnt cases are the worst; if they are not too badly hurt their sensibility is acute and they suffer dreadful agony. At about five o'clock the nurse begins to feel rather badly. She has to brace herself up and put on a big spurt to get through the mornings work, and perhaps at eight o'clock she will go to bed without her breakfast.

'A senior nurse's duties are somewhat different from those of the juniors. To begin with, she feels herself of some importance; she has charge of linen closets; she sees to the giving out of the food and gives out the medicines; when the doctors make rounds, if there is time she accompanies the head nurse; she makes herself acquainted with the state of the patients, and often has to be in charge of the ward.

'To anyone not initiated into the ways of medical men, giving out the medicines might mean a spoonful of something in a little water. A medicine list is an appalling undertaking at first - there may be thirty names on the list, some patients having as many as five or six different medicines; in fact, it practically amounts to one-dose prescriptions.

'Different quantities are given: drops, drachms, ounces, and so on. With some practice and with someone to take the medicines around quickly, a nurse can get through the list accurately in a remarkably short time, say fifteen to twenty minutes, but this is not often done; we usually take our time. (A nurse has learnt something of the properties and doses of the medicines in her class.)

'When a nurse has charge of a ward, or becomes a head nurse, any notions she may have had of her importance as a senior disappear. She feels herself responsible, and is responsible for the condition of the ward, the care of the patients, the instruction of the nurses, in fact for whatever is done or neglected. The doctors rely upon her for the faithful carrying out of their orders, and altogether she needs a good deal of judgment and tact.

'After receiving the notes of the night nurse and seeing that all the work is going on well, the head nurse goes round, note-book in hand, and inquires into the state of each patient; she questions them and listens to what they have to say; she also makes her own observations. In this way the nurse becomes acquainted with her patients, while she reports everything of note to the doctors.

There is an etiquette observed in the wards, but it is not very oppressive; the nurses on duty are subordinate to the doctors for the time being, and everything goes on with order and decorum. This may sound stiff and formal, but it is not so; it is only the fitness of things. We usually all work well together and there is seldom any friction.

The patients in Charity Hospital are the very poor of the city; some of them are only morally sick and needing a home; they puzzle the doctors to make a diagnosis. Most of their sickness, as we nurses know, has been brought on by overwork, poverty, drunkenness, laziness, and the like, but some are worthy and deserving persons.

'Often when a patient comes into the hospital she enters a moral atmosphere which is new to her. She is cleaned and made fairly comfortable; she has to drop many of her old habits of speech, and be a decent member of the hospital for the time being. If she is not too degraded she can see what is expected of her at once. We seldom have any trouble with the patients and rarely hear an improper word. A nurse never need submit to insubordination; on her complaint the patient is dismissed, but a very sick patient is seldom beyond endurance.

'They are often very witty, and if we are in the mood we can get lots of fun out of them. They are also very religious. They thank God for everything; everything is the will of God; their sickness, their troubles, their death; it never seems to occur to them that they might have a will of their own. In one way they have not much variety; they usually object to soap and water.

'As a rule the nurses are as good to the patients as they can be. Many of them remain in the hospital for a long time, and a nurse has the opportunity of showing them small kindnesses, perhaps writing a letter or giving them a garment or a few cents to pay their car fare. In those tedious cases of phthisis where the treatment is only palliative a nurse can be much to the patient.

The patients in the emergency hospitals are somewhat different; they are mostly of the mechanic class, and usually quite sick. That means business and getting them well, and they pass on. They are not so poor; they can even offer us money, either by way of bribe or reward. I heard of a nurse having the handsome sum of ten dollars offered to her, and I once came near having a pair of diamond ear-rings, only the patient changed his mind and would not undergo the operation.

The helpers spoken of in this sketch are women sentenced to the workhouse on Blackwell's Island for terms varying from three days to six months, and for such offences as drunkenness, vagrancy, and fighting in the streets. From the workhouse they are sent to do the scrubbing, laundry work, etc., in the institutions controlled by the Commissioners of Charities and Correction, who are obliged by law to use their labor. Most of them are the sodden, frowsy creatures who huddle into the prison van after the laconic ten days of the police justice, but they are all ages of bad eggs, as one of them once said to me, and taken together they form a curious class.

They are most punctilious in always speaking of each other as ladies, and the much-abused word is somewhat amusing when applied to a stout virago with a variegated eye.

Drunkenness, their common vice, and the cause of all their woe, is delicately alluded to as a weakness or a failing, and some of them seem rather proud of the number of times they have been sent up, while others regard it as the inevitable. Once I had to pass a woman who was scrubbing in a doorway at Charity, and as she moved her pail I recognized her and said,

'What, Mary, are you here again? I thought you weren't coming back.'

Her face fell as she answered,

'Yes, Maam, I thought so too,' and then she brightened up and said proudly, 'But it was the elegantest wake you ever see...'

Some of them again are decent and quiet enough when not possessed by the devil of drink, and it often happens that one of this better class will stay on as a helper after her sentence has expired, perhaps feeling that she is protected from herself while the river is between her and her boon companions, but sooner or later she is missing some day, she has gone over, and if she comes back it is in the prison boat.

Here follows the journal of an ordinary day at Charity Hospital, by one of the head-nurses:

Time: 7.30 A.M.

Scene: Ward 3, Medical.

Beds all unmade, a few patients up - these have faces washed and hair combed – the majority in bed with this duty still to be performed for them. A part of the floor at the front of the ward has been scrubbed. Mary, one of my prison helpers, is washing dishes at the table, and Bridget, the other, is taking soiled clothes from a large can and sorting them for the wash.

The atmosphere contains none too much oxygen; this can be explained by saying that the night-nurse is finishing her work in one of the other wards, and the patients in her absence have taken the precaution to close all of the windows for fear of taking cold. After giving an order for the windows to be let down, I take up the night notes and read:

Murphy: Died at 3 AM.

Ryan: Temperature, 1080; pulse, 120; respiration, 30. Antifebrin, grains iii., and other medicines given as ordered. Poultice applied last at 6 AM.

Patient passed a very restless night.

And so on, through the other cases in the ward. These notes are signed by the night nurse, who now comes in with the keys, looking pretty well fagged.

'Good-morning; I am sorry I have kept you waiting for the keys, but I have been so busy I could not get down sooner. Had a death in Ward 4, as well as the one here, and a patient in Ward 6 suffering from delirium tremens, besides the ordinary work.'

I now go over to where my assistants are putting on their caps and aprons and getting together the things necessary for work. Miss W. and Miss A. are here, but where is Miss H.? Miss W. answers:

'She was called up last night to go on the maternity service. The superintendent missed you, and asked me to tell you that another nurse could not be spared today.'

Oh, dear, thirty-two patients in the ward, and five of them so helpless that they have to be fed and cared for like babies, two pneumonia cases, and the usual number of phthisis and rheumatic subjects. Well, well, grumbling won't do the work, so we'll have to make the best of it.

Each of my assistants, armed with a pile of clean sheets and pillow-cases, proceeds to the lower end of the ward and commences the task of getting beds made, while I go to write the list of clothes for the laundry. Bridget counts the clothes while I stand by and take down the number of each of the different articles. This done, they are tied in large bundles and sent to the wash-house.

Now the medicines are to be given out. I measure and prepare them, while a convalescent patient carries them round to those in bed. My list is a long one, and it takes fully thirty-five minutes before they are all distributed, the bottles wiped off, and the medicine closet put in order. My next move is to take a list of medicines which need to be renewed, and leave it ready for the doctor's signature. It is now twenty-five minutes past eight, and Miss A. and Miss W. are making as good progress as possible at their respective sides; for it must be remembered that a nurse has often to stop what she is doing to attend to the wants of some particular patient, or to carry out an order if the time is due.

The railroad beds are still unmade. (A railroad bed is one that is unoccupied during the day, and therefore, as it were shunted and rolled out at night. They stand close together in the middle of the ward.) Occasionally we have a convalescent patient who can do this part of the work very well. We had one in this ward last week, but alas, for the frailty of human nature, she showed a disposition to quarrel with the other patients on very small pretexts, so she was dismissed. With a rueful thought of what might have been, I go to work at the beds. A patient goes ahead and strips them for me. We work with all our might and they are finished at ten minutes past nine. The side beds, too, are nearly finished. This part of the work necessarily takes much longer, as sick patients have to be placed in chairs and wrapped up in blankets, or, if they are too weak, lifted into other beds, so that their own can be made.

My next work is to take morning temperatures; when I have finished this, I see a large tin can standing near my table. It contains crackers, butter, eggs, and sugar. These have to be put away in their proper place, and the quantity noted. Now, I must write my diet-sheet, and order the supplies necessary for tomorrow. It is twenty-five minutes past nine, the beds are all made, the stands in order, the floor swept, and the table scrubbed.

The junior nurses are about through with washing faces and combing heads, and it is now high time that I should make a round of the ward and find out if there is any change in the patients condition to which the doctors attention should be called.

While this has been going on, the gruel and milk have been standing on the table, and the distribution of this falls to my share today also, as I have no senior nurse. Each bed-patient who cares for it is served with a portion on a tray; afterward the walking patients seat themselves at the table and take theirs. Now the doctors come in to make their morning visit, the house-doctor is told of any special complaints; he examines these patients, also any new ones who may not yet be under treatment, and leaves the new orders on my book.

While doing this work all morning, I have been trying to keep an eye on what my helpers are doing, and now take this time to make a thorough inspection of all parts of the ward, bathroom included. In the meantime the special diet has been divided among the patients needing it most. At eleven o'clock tonics are given out, afterward egg-nogs and milk-punches are made and distributed.

We now begin to breathe freely – the worst pressure is over if we get no new patients. Our hopes along that line are doomed to disappointment, for the helpers from the women's bath-room now announce the arrival of two new patients, and Miss W. disappears to superintend their bathing.

I am congratulating myself on not having a stretcher case at any rate, when two men come in with one. Miss A. quickly places screens round a bed, and a rubber sheet over the clean bedclothes. The woman is lifted on the bed, and her temperature, pulse, etc., taken. Her own clothes are soon removed, and a warm sponge-bath given and hair combed. These operations have effected a wonderful change in her appearance, and she now looks a little more like a Caucasian, whereas, before the bath, she might have belonged to one of the darker races of mankind.

The doctor is notified that there are three new patients in the ward. It is twelve o'clock; Miss A. and I go to dinner, and leave Miss W. to superintend the patient's noonday meal, and give out medicines afterward. We return at one o'clock, and Miss W. goes, with the right to remain off duty till four o'clock.

The ward is now to be swept again and put in order for the afternoon. This is hardly accomplished when two huge bundles of clothes are carried in, and in ten minutes time two more. These have to be sorted and counted. Before we proceed to the folding of them the afternoon milk and other extras are given out. That done and the table cleared, we fold the clothes as quickly as we can. In due time this is finished, Miss A. is making a poultice in the bath-room, and I am putting the clothes in the closet, when someone calls 'Nurse, nurse!' I turn to see where the sound comes from, and notice several patients pointing to a bed in the far corner of the ward.

I hurry down and find the patients clothes saturated with blood- a hemorrhage from the lungs. Screens are immediately placed around the bed, cracked ice given, and the doctor summoned. He comes at once, the flow of blood seems to have ceased, medicine is ordered, and the doctor goes. The patient's clothes are now changed very carefully, and she is made as comfortable as possible. The screens are just put away when another stretcher is brought in, and Miss W., who has now returned, gives the usual treatment.

It is time for the afternoon tonics, and eggnogs and punches are again distributed; after this I take advantage of a few spare minutes to enter the names and addresses of patients in a book kept for the purpose. Discharged patients are also marked off.

The patients have supper between half-past four and five. At hall-past five, Miss A. retires from the ward, the remaining time till half-past seven being hers to rest. In the meantime, the doctor has been in and left a few orders.

The giving out of the evening medicines falls to me, while Miss W. attends to the patients needs in other ways. If I had a fourth nurse, I might be relieved from duty; but it cannot be thought of now. This is the evening for carbolizing the side beds; the helpers do this, while we follow and restore things to order. The rest of the time till hall-past seven is spent in making patients comfortable for the night, and writing down new orders and notes on the patients' condition for the night nurse. We are quite willing to deliver her the keys when she comes in, and bid her goodnight, while we go home tired enough to sleep soundly.

Charity Hospital, as I have said, has chiefly chronic cases. The work in the accident or emergency hospitals is somewhat different, as will be seen by the following notes:

Leaving the Island at 7 a.m., after three-quarters of an hour's ride in boat and car, I reach Gouverneur Hospital. On my arrival I receive from the night nurse both a verbal and written account of all that has happened of importance during the night - arrival of new patients, serious symptoms which may have developed in certain cases, new orders which have been given by the doctor, or old ones which may have been countermanded, etc.

Then begins the work of the day. The ward is thoroughly scrutinized, to discover little things which the helpers are apt to do slightingly, or not to do at all; stands are dusted, clean covers and curtains put on, if necessary; every patient and bed must undergo thorough inspection.

Everything is done as quickly as possible, for the visiting may be looked for at any time after 9 a.m., and it is the ambition of each nurse to have her ward spotlessly clean.

I have six pneumonia cases, who are poulticed regularly every three hours; they are also kept on milk diet, and, of course, require particular attention. I have just finished putting on my last poultice when the visiting comes in, followed by the house surgeons, senior and junior. I accompany them to the different beds, ready to receive all orders, and impart any information which may be required of me.

During the rounds of the physicians, an ambulance call is given; in due time the man is carried in on a stretcher; I rush to prepare a bed, which consists in turning down the covers, and protecting the whole with a rubber sheet; with the assistance of one of the helpers the patient is placed in bed. It proves to be a poisoning case. As quick as possible I get ready pitchers of tepid water, a pail, and a stomach-pump. The doctor then begins his operations, and I stand near to assist him. If the patient is very weak, I administer stimulants hypodermically; an emetic is given. Fortunately, the case has been attended to in time, and is soon out of all immediate danger, although very weak.

A little boy has been brought in with hand and wrist literally pulverized; the poor little fellows cries are heartrending; an anesthetic is administered, I carefully sponge the blood away from the injured parts, get ready the different solutions, gauzes, bandages, splints, etc., and stand near to assist in any way that I can. (I took care of the little boy for six weeks after that, and he was sent home cured, having lost but two fingers.)

Standing by, awaiting his turn is a stonecutter. He must have taken his thumb for a stone, for he has simply hammered it off. The compression of his lips and the pallor of his face give evidence of the pain he is suffering. A thin piece of skin on one side keeps the thumb from being entirely severed from the hand; the doctor replaces it and sews it on, but eventually, to save the hand, it had to be amputated.

Fortunately there are no more accident cases on hand, and I am free once more to attend to my other patients. I give out the three-hour medicines, renew my poultices, and take the temperature, pulse, and respiration of a patient who came in about an hour ago; but, finding his temperature normal, I let him remain seated until the doctor comes in.

After dinner I give out the noon medicines, examine the beds of the helpless patients, and find out from them if there is anything I can do to add to their comfort. After attending to their wants, and performing numberless duties which it would be impossible to relate, I finally feel satisfied that every patient has been made comfortable; then I tear up bandages, which are given to the convalescent patients to roll; prepare solutions and different kinds of gauzes to be used during operations; in the meantime keeping a watchful eye on all around, so that no patient shall suffer from want of attention.

About 4 p.m. I have to take the temperature, pulse, and respiration of each patient, which, in a ward where there are twenty, takes quite a length of time. After the temperatures are taken, I see that each patient has his supper, then write an account of all the orders I have received, which are to be continued during the night, renew the poultices, give out the medicines, see that the ward is in perfect order, and am relieved at 6p.m. by the night nurse.

Account of a Night at Hospital
By a Gouverneur Night Nurse, 1890

The following is an account of the routine of a night at Gouverneur Hospital:

'The night nurse of Gouverneur does not often arise with bright face and laughing eye, feeling as fresh and happy as a lark, at half-past four in the afternoon of a hot July day, but she scrambles out of bed and dons the stripes as quickly as possible, that she may not be late for the dinner at five o'clock. At six, we get to the wards to relieve the day nurses from duty, and are often greeted with,

'Well, I think you will have rather a hard night.'

'As I look around the ward I find the man in the first bed is a sunstroke case, with a temperature of 105, and the orders are to keep ice-bags on head and abdomen, give ice-baths, and take temperature every fifteen minutes until the temperature falls below 102. The child in the corner has pneumonia and has on a jacket poultice of linseed-meal, which must be changed as often as it becomes cold, and the child watched very closely. The delirious patient in the other corner is to have an ice-cap on his head, which must be kept well filled with cracked ice. He has a fracture of the base of the skull, and he raves and shouts most of the night.

'We have two patients more than we have beds, consequently we must prepare four patients to be transferred to Bellevue, in order to have beds for the patients who will come in during the night.

'At nine o'clock the doctors make their rounds, and oftentimes there are dressings that the doctor has had no time to do during the day, and the nurse must always be ready to wait upon the doctor the moment he enters the ward.

At eleven o'clock, there is an ambulance call and a man is brought in with three stab wounds. He is covered with blood, hands, face, and clothing, has a long wound on the face, a deep one in the shoulder, and a small one in the abdomen. The wounds are sewed and dressings put on. These dressings are scarcely finished, when there comes another call, and the ambulance brings in this time a fine-looking young man with a deep wound in the forearm. From his nervous tremor and restlessness I conclude he has been drinking heavily, and this is confirmed when the house surgeon gives the order for a half-ounce of the IDT mixture immediately.

His wound is dressed, and he is launched into bed and tied down. Presently he begins to see snakes and all sorts of creeping things upon his bed, and he wants to get up and eat the man in the bed next him. He finally becomes so violent that he is put into handcuffs and taken to the alcoholic cells at Bellevue.

Then things quiet down for perhaps an hour, which time must be devoted to the man with sunstroke and the child with pneumonia. These, however, have not been wholly neglected, for there was time to make a poultice for the child, and the helper has attended to the bathing of the man, whose temperature has fallen only one and one-half degree.

Now it is time to begin the morning's work of the wards, for they must be all in order for the day nurse when she comes on duty at eight o'clock. The temperature, pulse, and respiration of each patient in the wards must be taken and noted upon the chart, also any new treatment ordered during the night, and anything noteworthy in the condition of the patient. Each bed is to be made, bed-linen and patients clothing to be changed, if soiled, while the floors are swept and washed by the helpers.

The medicines are given out at various times through the night, as each becomes due. Then there is the patient's breakfast to look after, and to see that all are served who may eat the food, and that those who are on special diet may get nothing but that allowed them, whatever it may be.

It would certainly seem that these women earn ten or even fifteen dollars a month besides their board and lodging.

Account of a serious operation from a Nurse's point of view
By a Theatre Nurse, 1890

The nurse is responsible for making antiseptic everything connected with an operation, except the surgical instruments. She prepares the room, has the floor and paint scrubbed, and every table washed with antiseptic solution. The dressings are most scrupulously prepared, being boiled and soaked and wrapped in antiseptic towels, or kept until needed in large glass jars. The nurse is further responsible for having everything in the room which the surgeon may possibly want, such as hot water, ice, hot-water bottles, stimulants, etc., and must be prepared for every emergency which, during the operation, may possibly arise.

The patient is prepared by the nurse, who gives a full bath, braids the hair, puts on clean and suitable clothing, and arranges her on the table, where she is always covered with a sheet or a single blanket if necessary. Another nurse helps the doctor give the anesthetic, and in fact, there are usually three nurses at an operation of any importance, the head-nurse being in charge and the other two her aids. She herself keeps her best eye on the operator and stands in a certain place where she can readily hand him hot towels, sponges, bowls of solution, anything he may need. The second nurse watches the supply of hot towels, solutions, sponges, hot and cold water, etc., while the third helps the junior doctor who is etherizing the patient, and fetches and carries, i.e., empties out water and puts it outside the door, where some patient is stationed to carry it away and fill up empty pitchers. In running an operation a nurse always aims at having it go off without a hitch, and sometimes it does, sometimes not.

Occasionally an operator is unreasonable and asks for the moon, and occasionally he makes a mistake and loses his head, and then the nurses have a poor time of it, being blamed if they have no boiling-hot beef-tea or brandy when there is no means of heating it in the room, the operation having already lasted over an hour. A doctor, if he is a gentleman, usually thanks the nurse after a long operation, and then she feels like doing anything for him.

Their hard day over, the nurses go to the Home, which is the stone building at the south end of Blackwell's Island. There they have a comfortable sitting-room with books and magazines and ledge (there is no superfluous furniture)- and a piano, and in summer they can play lawn tennis outside, or rest and watch the crowd of boats that is always going up and down the great river.

But all the evenings are not given to amusements, except during July and August. The school is divided into junior, senior, and graduating classes, and each has a quiz or lesson once a week, and sometimes oftener, which is usually taught by the Assistant Superintendent. A skeleton, some large colored diagrams, and a manikin who is represented as if he were skinned, which gives him an unpleasant likeness to Marsyas or St. Bartholomew, and who takes to pieces in a startling manner, are much used at these lessons, while some of the physicians and surgeons of the visiting staff give lectures to the classes from time to time.

When at last the two years course is over, a board of physicians hold the final examination which a nurse must pass before receiving her diploma.

At private nursing, a woman receives from $15 to $25 a week, which would pay her well if she were always busy; but she is subject to be overworked for some months and idle for several more, and an excellent nurse said recently that she should be satisfied to be sure of making $600 a year.

There are signs that the market is beginning to be overstocked. The four large schools which I have already spoken of have already 911 graduates and every hospital of whatever size must now have its training - school, so that each year brings a new crop of certificated nurses, more or less trained, according to their capacity and opportunities.

Some of the schools announce that they have many more applicants than they can take, from which outsiders have naturally been led to conclude that pupils would be willing to come without pay, but the superintendents, who are already feeling the effects of competition, know well that any such move would be fatal to a really high standard.

This competition between the schools has not been without good results, in that it has stimulated the different boards in charge of them to greater efforts in the direction of comfort in the Homes, and a distinct and attractive course of instruction; and it is to be hoped that something may be done toward shortening the long hours of work in the wards.

In regard to graduates, the time has come when the profession, if it is to be such, must be protected. This can best be done by the formation of a central committee or board, which shall recognize only graduates of standard schools, shall take the testimony of their superintendents as to the fitness and trust-worthiness of such graduates, and after submitting them to an examination, shall give them a degree or diploma not obtainable in any other way.

The law sets the standard for physicians by recognizing only the degrees of certain colleges, which might be difficult in the case of training-schools, but something must be done to indicate and to protect the women who have earned the best right to live by their trade. It is not enough to let the stronger crowd out the weaker, as in the case of stenographers or telegraph operators, because doctors have learnt to expect intelligent help from a trained nurse, and if she fail them in a critical case, it may mean the difference between life and death.

Mary Cadwalader Jones, November, 1890

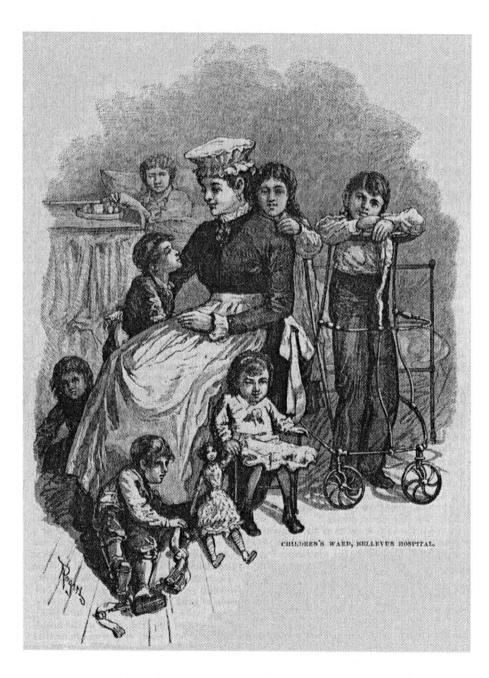

Children's Ward, Bellevue Hospital

CHAPTER FIVE

A Nurse Should Be...

(Editor's Note: although this item was originally written and published in the UK, it was republished in the USA a number of years later as an important reference source and example for American nurses to follow)

Every physician recognizes the importance of good nursing. In the treatment of disease, medicinal agents are necessary to combat the various symptoms as they arise, but it is equally important that the surroundings of the patient should be so arranged that he may be supported and tided over the critical period of his illness. It is not too much to say that in many illnesses good nursing is more than half the battle. When a man is seriously ill he is practically as helpless as a child, and can neither think nor act for himself. He is fortunate should there be some friend or relative who will take the initiative for him, but there are many people - often men in good social position - who have no one about them whom they would care to trust. The sick man sends for his doctor, and nurses are provided on whom rests the responsibility of seeing that he is properly cared for, and that no advantage is taken of his helplessness. The trust is a sacred one, and for the honour of the nursing community is rarely or never abused.

By a sort of tacit understanding, nursing is generally, we may say almost universally, regarded as a woman's vocation. It is very desirable that the nurse should be a young woman, and both in hospital and private practice, women are employed both in the female and in the male wards. There are, it is true, men who adopt nursing as a calling, but compared with the women they are few in number. The so-called 'male nurse' partakes more of the nature of the valet or attendant than of the nurse proper. In exception-al cases where a patient is extremely violent and cannot be controlled in any other way, the services of a man may be found necessary, but practical experience shows that a delirious patient is far more likely to be quieted by the gentle touch of a female hand than by any mere exhibition of physical strength. Whilst recognising the occasional utility of a man as a nurse we are inclined to think that the occupation is one which is more safely left in the hands of women. The following remarks apply almost entirely to the female sick-nurse, and are not applicable to the male attendant, or to the nurse or nursemaid who is entrusted with the care of healthy children.

Social Status of the Nurse

The social status of the sick-nurse has undergone many curious changes during the last twenty or thirty years. Thirty years or so ago a trained nurse was a rarity, and when sickness broke out in a family the patient was usually nursed by a relative with the assistance of an old servant or a superannuated charwoman.

Even in our large general hospitals, the state of affairs was not very much better, and the nursing staff consisted chiefly of uneducated women who, however well-intentioned, were practically untrained. They were in the main honest and trustworthy, the only serious charge that could be brought against them being that they were addicted to the use of spirits, and had a constant habit of sampling the patient's whisky or brandy.

Suddenly a marvellous change took place; the old-fashioned nurse was ousted from her position, and nursing was raised to the dignity of a 'profession.' It was the popular fad of the day, and women all over the country became 'nursing mad.' They abandoned their household duties and eagerly sought for admittance into the various training establishments. They donned more or less appropriate costumes, and astonished their stay-at-home sisters by the facility with which they employed abstruse medical terms, and by their gruesome stories of the horrors of the operating room and wards.

Their enthusiasm was so great that they willingly paid heavy premiums for instruction, taking little care to ascertain whether it was good, bad, or indifferent. The demand created a supply, and nursing institutions of all kinds sprang up all over the country, some of them undoubtedly supplying a want, but many of them serving simply to bring grist to the mills of their astute promoters. Although the system was, no doubt, in many respects faulty, the result was beneficial in this sense: that nurses of high character and of admitted competence were to be obtained without difficulty.

Of late, however, there has been a decided reaction, and nursing can no longer be regarded as a lucrative calling. It has to a very great extent ceased to be fashionable, and so far the change is not to be regretted. There are those, however, who hint that the *moral* of the class as a whole does not stand on quite so high a level as before the reaction set in.

Such critics account for the retrogression which they believe themselves to have observed partly by the fact that the market is over-crowded, and that constant work is difficult to obtain, and partly by the fact that the nurse is accorded an amount of liberty which is somewhat unusual in the case of other young women.

When she has completed her training and leaves the hospital, she may commence nursing on her own account, and in these circumstances, when she is not actually fulfilling an engagement, she is from the nature of the case under no supervision. Such critics would certainly admit that in the vast majority of instances the emancipation from control leads to no abuse, while, on the other hand, those who hold that the criticisms are ill-founded will not deny that such freedom as this may not be altogether unattended with danger.

On the whole, however, the modern nurse thoroughly merits the high estimation in which she is held, and it goes without saying that in the ranks of the sisterhood may be found characters of the very highest type. No one can assert that the average nurse is not faithful and attentive in the performance of her duties, and the severest of her censors will concede that she is an immense improvement on the nurse of thirty years ago. It is almost an insult to her, indeed, to mention the two types in the same sentence.

<u>The Nurse's Qualification</u>

The qualifications required to be a successful nurse are necessarily of a high order, and this applies not only to the trained nurse, but to her embryo sister who wishes to adopt nursing as a calling.

In the first place she must be not only physically, but constitutionally strong. She must be not only well formed, but must have certain powers of resistance. A girl, for example, who is subject to sick headaches, or who readily 'knocks up,' will never make a good nurse. The best type of nursing girl is one who is tall and strong, and who has a certain suppleness of movement.

One who is accustomed to play lawn-tennis, who can ride, and skate, and row, makes the best material. If she can dance, especially if she is an enthusiastic dancer, it is a great advantage, for graceful carriage is a thing to be cultivated, and nothing is more distasteful in a sick-room than a suspicion of clumsiness. If in addition to being well-formed she is favoured with good looks, it is all in her favour, for doctors readily recognise the influence of an attractive person in the management of refractory patients.

A nurse who aspires to rise in her profession should have a soft and evenly modulated voice, for harsh notes jar on the ears of sensitive patients. With regard to her general education, she must be able to speak her own language correctly, and if she has a smattering of French and German so much the better. She should be able to write a good hand, and should have an elementary knowledge of how to keep accounts.

Respecting her moral attributes, it may be said that a girl who has been brought up in a country parsonage, and has had little experience of the world, is hardly fitted for hospital work. In the wards, she will be brought in constant contact with people of various modes of thought, and if she is unable to adapt herself to her surroundings, her novitiate will of necessity be a very uncomfortable one.

It is true that the embryo nurse rapidly acquires knowledge, but if she has strong views and prejudices she will soon find that her life is not and easy one. This is still more the case in private practice, for people when they are ill are not tolerant of opinions which are not in accordance with their own. A nurse has to learn the very useful lesson that she is not a reformer of other people's morals, and that her highest claim to consideration and respect is that she carries out her duties conscientiously.

Nursing should not be undertaken from sentimental motives, or, from any notion of becoming one of the 'Guardian Angels' of the novelist. Such an idea will assuredly end in disappointment, for it will be found that the really sick have but a poor appreciation of sentiment, that the routine duties of the sick-room are monotonous and tiresome, and leave but scant time for indulging one's imagination or poetic feelings.

It is hardly necessary to say that a nurse should be honest and truthful, for the vast majority of English nurses possess these qualifications in the very highest degree. When a man living alone, say in chambers, is suddenly taken ill, he must of necessity be nursed, almost equally of necessity the nurse has to be given charge, not only of his expenditure, but of his personal effects.

The nurse is commonly a perfect stranger to him, and although this responsibility arises in thousands of cases we have never heard of a single instance in which the slightest suspicion of dishonesty or unfair dealing has arisen. The only danger to the patient is entirely of another character, for it sometimes happens that the invalid during his long period of convalescence, becomes so enamoured of his kindly attendant that he finds it impossible to dispense with her services, and marries her!

Amateur Nurses

There is a decided prejudice against amateur nurses, but if there is a young woman in the house who is willing to learn, it is astonishing how quickly she can be taught by a doctor who is accustomed to teaching, and who has those personal characteristics which are so essential for the formation of good pupils. If the doctor will teach, and the pupil is intelligent and willing, a very serviceable nurse may be improvised in a few hours. There is no particular mystery about nursing, and the technicalities are easily acquired. If the raw material is there it can be knocked into shape very readily. In cases of emergency, it is wonderful how much can be accomplished by a little mutual good understanding.

Relatives always make worse nurses than those who have no such tie to the patient, especially if they have had no previous training. They cannot be expected to regard with the necessary calmness the suffering of one to whom they are tied by bonds of friendship and consanguinity, and there is nothing more trying to an invalid to see constantly around his bed the too-anxious countenances of his family, the doleful expressions of which are often the cause of a needless and mischievous sensation of alarm. Again, relatives have not the necessary control over patients; and one often sees the strength of an invalid wasted by little peevish family squabbles over food or medicine, which would have been taken without question if offered to him by a nurse with authority on her side.

Invalid children are proverbially naughty and perverse with their parents, and invalid parents are usually unwilling to be controlled by their children.

Training

A young woman who wishes to be trained as a nurse usually applies to the lady superintendent of one of the nursing homes connected with a London or provincial hospital. She is furnished with a code of rules and regulations, and is required to sign an agreement before being admitted as a probationer.

This agreement is often of a very stringent and arbitrary nature, and it is never safe to enter into such an engagement without first submitting the document to a solicitor or a business friend. If any objection is offered to this course it may be pretty safely assumed that the contract is of such a nature that it will not bear investigation. It must be remembered that it is not the hospital which undertakes to train nurses, and that the nursing establishment is merely a trading concern, which has an agreement to provide the hospital with a certain number of nurses at a price.

The nursing institutions are not in any way charitable bodies, and do no gratuitous work, so that they have no real claim on the public. They sometimes appeal for support on the ground that they nurse the sick-poor in our hospitals, but they are liberally paid for their services, and have many privileges given them. Some of them are not above 'sweating' the nurses, and derive a handsome profit from the transaction. They pay the nurse from (say) £16 to £30 or so a year, according to her proficiency, and do not hesitate to charge from two to three guineas a week for her services.

The age at which a nurse should begin her training is a matter concerning which there is some difference of opinion. One authority thinks that the best age is between twenty-five and thirty. This is an entire mistake, for a person who attempts to enter a business or profession at the age of thirty rarely does much at it. Twenty-one is a good age to begin, and forty is a good age at which to retire. A woman is much older than a man at the age of forty, and by that time a woman should have made some permanent provision in life for herself. Few doctors will employ old nurses, and few patients care to have them.

At most hospitals, paying probationers are received. The charge varies from £30 a year to a guinea a week. Non-paying probationers are considered to be proficient at the expiration of twelve months. They are usually required to sign an agreement containing a clause, that 'during the three years succeeding the completion of their training, they will enter into service as hospital or infirmary nurses in such situations as may from time to time be procured for them by the committee.' On inquiry, it will often be found that 'the committee' is not the committee of the hospital, but the committee of the nursing home.

The nurse's wages vary somewhat in different institutions, but in all they are small. For example, at St. Bartholomew's Hospital they are £8, £12, £20, and £30 for probationers, while staff nurses are paid £35 and £40; at King's College Hospital the wages are none the first year, £15 the second year, £20 the third year, £30 the fourth year, £33 the fifth year, and £36 the sixth year; at the Paddington Green Hospital for Children the wages are £12 for the first year and £14 for the second, while nurses are paid from £25 to £36, and sisters from £30 to £40.

In some of the regulations, we note that the nurses 'pay their own laundry.' In one institution it is stated that there is 'an allowance of two shillings a week for washing,' a sum which is certainly inadequate. As a rule indoor uniform, or material for making up the uniform, is provided after the end of the trial month, but in some hospitals there is no such provision during the first year of probationership. Outdoors uniform is seldom provided.

In some of the agreements there is a clause to the effect that 'probationers will be subject to be discharged at any time by the matron in case of misconduct, or should she consider them inefficient or negligent of their duties.' The expression 'at any time' seems to imply that the probationer may be dismissed at a moment's notice. Nothing is said about any right of appeal to the managing committee, and the matron is evidently entrusted with full powers.

The hours of duty for nurses vary somewhat in different hospitals. In the regulations of one hospital we find the following note:- 'Hours on duty, twelve; two and a half hours off duty every alternate day, and half a day once a month.' At another hospital the hours on duty are given as twelve. At a third the day nurses rise at 6 a.m. and retire to rest at 10 p.m., but they are allowed an hour and a half for exercise in the middle of the day.

At Guy's Hospital, the holidays are two weeks at the end of the first year, three weeks at the end of the second, and afterwards four weeks. Staff nurses get five weeks, and sisters the same, and also every alternate Sunday to Monday.

The regulations for the most part show an improvement upon those that obtained a few years ago, though in some cases it is still true that they are drawn up too much in the interest of the training school, and with too little regard to the welfare of the nurses and probationers. One advantage which nurses now enjoy is that conferred upon them by the Royal National Pension Fund for Nurses. In many hospitals all the nurses who join this excellent Fund have half the premium paid for them by the institution.

The Nurse's Dress

The nurse must be cleanly in her person, both for her own safety and for the sake of those with whom she comes in contact. Her dress should be simple, but by all means let it be becoming. Many ladies who take to nursing think it necessary to assume the most hideous garb imaginable. If the exigencies of religion necessitate this course, we regret our inability to argue the case, but on medical grounds we feel quite sure that the dress of an attendant on the sick should be simple and becoming, and not such as will excite the wonder, the fear, or the risibility of a patient.

The dress should be just long enough to clear the ground, and should be made of printed calico, or some other *washing material* of a light colour and a smooth surface. Moreover, it should be frequently washed. Some of the nursing sisterhoods adopt a robe made of black flannel with long hanging sleeves. Nothing can be imagined more ill-suited for a nurse's dress. The blackness of it prevents the ready detection of dirt, the rough surface and absorbent texture is ready to catch and suck up all disease particles, whether dry or liquid, and the dangling sleeves and floating stole and girdle are certainly likely to hitch in every projecting object, and as they fulfil no useful purpose, it is difficult to see why they should be retained. Some of these lugubrious dresses are worn, too, for as long a period as were the hair shirts of the mediaeval hermits. We have heard a sister boasting of the grimy penance to which she had subjected herself for more than six months.

It is to be regretted that ladies who perform their duties with so much zeal and with the highest possible intelligence, should run the risk of marring much of the effect of their good deeds by adhering to a fashion of dress which ought to have died out with the Middle Ages, and before the dawning of the science of hygiene.

A nurse should wear a neat cap, and should be careful to have shoes which do not creak. A pair of scissors and a pin-cushion carried from a girdle will be found also of the greatest service. It is customary with many nurses to carry with them a small pocket case filled with instruments, such as scissors, dressing forceps, caustic holder, tongue depressor, and so forth, but these things are intended only for show, and are quite unnecessary.

The Nurse's Outfit

A nurse requires some kind of an outfit, but it need be of the most inexpensive description. A clinical thermometer in a metal case can be obtained for 2s., scissors with blunt or sharp points are 2s. 6d. a pair, a grooved director with scoop costs 1s. 9., and a silver probe with an eye or sharp point 1s. If the nurse chooses to indulge in the luxury of a case or wallet, she can get it complete, filled with a variety of instruments, for 19s. 6d., and can have her name stamped on it in gold letters for 1s. extra.

'Silent shoes' for use in the sick room are a little bit more expensive, but are supplied by most bootmakers at a price ranging from 6s. 6d. to 10s. 6d.

Examination for Nurses

At many hospitals, nurses are required to pass examinations. We have had an opportunity of inspecting some examination papers, and we must admit that some of the questions do not impress us with a sense of their utility. We give one or two examples:-

1. What is meant by (a) hydrocarbon diet, and (b) diabetic diet? Explain something of the principles on which these diet tables are constructed in relation to the diseases for which they are prescribed.

2. Describe in full the principles of central galvanisation.

Such questions as these as applied to the training of nurses, are not only useless, but border on the farcical. In a recent work on nursing which deals with the practical side of the question, we find the following commonsense view of the subject, which we commend to the so-called 'authorities' of nursing establishments:-'Instead of a nurse leaning over a bed and holding the cup of cooling drink to the fevered lips, we have a vision before us of a frantic probationer with her fingers in her ears bent double over a dirty old copy of Kirke's 'Handbook of Physiology', and the second picture is as true as the first.'

Hospital Life

There is good reason for supposing that in some of our hospitals, the food and sleeping accommodation for nurses are still not what they ought to be. A few years ago a commission was appointed with the view of investigating this question, but many of the nurses, although evidently holding strong views on the subject, declined to afford any information, being afraid of offending the authorities. One nurse wrote:- 'I am sure, from what I have heard, that the matron would not wish me to begin joining in the discussion now made public, and knowing so well her views on the subject, I think it would be neither loyal nor right to take, in ever so small a way, a part in the matter.´

Sentiments such as these are in a sense praise-worthy, and reflect much credit on the writer, but at the same time it must be remembered that a hospital is a public institution supported for the most part by voluntary contributions, and that those who contribute their money have a perfect right to inquire into the truth of rumours, and that the proper feeding of the nurses is as much a matter for concern and, if necessary, public investigation, as the care and welfare of the patients themselves. A public institution should have nothing to hide, and if there is a suspicion of abuse, the sooner the wrong is righted the better for all concerned. If people will not help themselves, it is hardly likely that others will do it for them.

Some nurses, however, were not so reticent, and expressed their views freely and in no measured terms. One of them wrote:- 'At times the cooking has been very bad, quite spoiling and wasting the food.' Another said:- 'A little more attention to the cooking and serving of the food would render it much more appetising without additional expense. The monotony of the diet and not the quality is distasteful to the tired nurse.'

The *Lancet*, commenting on these statements said, 'This is obviously a very serious grievance, and one, moreover, that need not exist at all. An efficient cook is much less expensive than an inefficient one, for bad cooking means waste.'

The fact is that a large hospital is a very complex institution. What is the business of many people seems to be the business of no one. In the first place, there is the cook with a staff of subordinates. The cook is responsible to the steward, and the steward is responsible to the secretary, who, in his turn, is responsible to the house committee which meets once a week and is appointed at the annual meeting of the governors.

The house committee is usually composed of a number of individuals who are personally actuated by the very best principles; but the majority of whom know little or nothing about household management, and despise such trivialities as good cooking. If the house committee does not move the secretary, he naturally enough does not move them, for as a salaried official, he prefers a life of peace and quietness, and endeavours to make things work smoothly.

The nurses themselves are not organised, and are under the thumb of the matron, who promptly suppresses any expression of discontent. If any individual nurse were to take action, and appeal to the house committee, she would receive very little support, and would probably be told that she was 'not strong enough for the work.'

The resident staff of the hospital - the house physicians and the house surgeons- are as a rule none too well fed, but they are in constant touch with the permanent staff of the hospital, and have a habit of expressing themselves strongly and effectively if their wants are not attended to. They are a fearless body of young men, who have before now been known to champion the cause of the nurses, and make a strong fight on their behalf.

Whatever difference of opinion there may be respecting the feeding of the nurses, there can be no doubt that in nearly all our hospitals they are disgracefully overworked. The universal custom is to have only two 'shifts' in the twenty-four hours, so that each nurse is on duty for about twelve hours at a time.

As a matter of fact, the nurse rarely goes off duty the moment she is relieved, as she has to make up her report and hand over her instructions for the care of the patients to her successor, so that it not uncommonly happens that her twelve hours are extended to thirteen.

The twelve hours' system, as need hardly be said, is a cruel strain on the strength and nerve of a woman. One nurse who was interviewed on the subject said:

'In my opinion, the chief evil of the present system of nursing is the long hours the nurses are compelled to be on their feet, and there will be no remedy for that until the day is divided into three parts of eight hours with three relays of nurses. The night nurses are especially hard worked, for they are on duty twelve hours, and in the medical wards often have not the chance of sitting down even for half an hour; then after a hard night they have beds to make, washing of patients, dusting, and breakfast to prepare and to give to each patient.'

Another says, 'Fourteen hours of work, which not only includes hard manual, but also responsible and anxious work, is, I consider, too much for any woman. I have now worked in a hospital for over a year, and my experience is that the whole cry of nurses off duty is, 'Oh ! I am so tired! Should this be? Should a nurse off duty feel so worn out as she does? I quite think that the eight hours' system should be introduced in hospitals. Why should not some little bit of the charity which is so freely given to the patients be extended to the nurses?'

Another very decided grievance is the shortness of the annual holiday. The allowance in some instances is two weeks for a probationer, three for a staff nurse, and four for a 'sister.' A probationer in one hospital where the leave of absence is only ten days in the year, says,

'The committee will not hear of our having a longer one. When one spends two days in the train, as some of us have to do, it leaves us with eight days, and to spend about £3 on it seems waste.'

Considering that the poor girl's salary would in all probability be no more than £16 a year, her complaint is not altogether an unreasonable one. The difficulty would be easily overcome by slightly overstaffing the nursing department, instead of understaffing it, as is so commonly the case in even our most wealthy institutions. Those who wish to see the moral tone of the sisterhood rise above its present high level should exert themselves to ensure that they are not overworked and underfed, and that they are allowed reasonable time for rest and recreation.

Year after year, many promising young women break down and abandon their calling, and it is strange, all things considered, that the number of those who take to other employments is not even greater.

Nurse's Accommodation

The difficulty of accommodating a nurse in a small household is often very great. She must have a bedroom, and often enough there is no room to spare. She, of course, must never be asked to take her meals with the servants, and should either dine with the family, or what is better, should have her meals sent to her own room. She cannot be expected to be always on duty, and in a severe case two nurses are absolutely necessary. When the nurse has finished her 'turn,' she is at liberty to do just as she likes, and may go to bed or go out as she thinks best.

If she dines with the family the patient's condition should not be made a subject of discussion. The best way is to treat the nurse, not only well and kindly, but liberally. She is always better for change of scene and recreation, and if, when she is off duty, she elects to go to a place of amusement or to enjoy herself in any other way, no possible objection can be offered, provided only that she does not put other people to inconvenience.

Wearing of Uniform

A nurse in the sick-room wears her nurse's dress, but it is open to question whether she should appear in the streets in that guise. Some people have a decided objection to seeing a nurse in uniform leaving their house, and their wishes in this respect must be observed. A few years ago, it was common enough to see persons parading the streets in nursing dress whose connection with nursing was of the slightest. Those were the days when a good many young ladies were coquetting with the nurse's vocation. Now it may safely be assumed that the nurse's uniform is not worn without proper warrant. At some hospitals there is an understanding that the nurse wears uniform only when actually on duty.

Nurses' Gossip

A nurse must not talk. We do not mean by this that a nurse is to abstain from holding conversation with a chronic invalid, but we wish our caution to apply particularly to those who have the care of acute invalids, to whom talking is an effort, and with whom anything like argument is quite out of place.

If food or medicine is to be given, let the portion or the dose be prepared, and when ready offer it to the patient as if there no question that he were going to take it. Never say; 'Will you take this, or try that?' or, 'Shall I get your medicine now?' or put similar questions.

There is no use in doing it, and if the invalid raise objections, as is often the case, the necessity for argument arises, which is a thing always to be avoided. Inexperienced nurses are very apt to pester and bother a patient with incessant sympathetic questionings, 'Are you in pain now, dear?' 'Does your head ache?' 'Are you lying comfortably?' 'Will you have the door open?' and so forth. This is bad. The good nurse watches her patient, and is quick to detect any complaint or sign of discomfort, but her sympathy manifests itself in some action designed to remedy what is amiss, rather than in misplaced expressions of pity.

Some nurses worry their patients almost to distraction by talking about their 'cases.' Most patients object very strongly to having nursing or medical papers brought into their rooms, and as a rule they take very little interest in hospitals and details of operations.

Nurses, from the peculiarity of their relations to their patients, often become possessed of information regarding them which ought to be considered perfectly sacred, never to be breathed to human ear. Happily the cases are few in which the temptation to tell a secret overcomes the sense of honour, and so these private matters become the conversation of gossiping women.

Nothing must be withheld from the doctor that can affect the patient's interest, but the nurse should never speak of her patient except in that general way which can hurt no one, and even then, with this exception, she should take care not to indulge in what is called 'harmless gossip.'

Many people consider they may ask questions of nurses about their patients which they would not dare to ask the sick person or his friends. Nurses must be on their guard not to be led to say anything which, were they in the patient's place, they would not like said of themselves. Many people - women particularly - are selfish from want of thought, rather than from want of heart, and many women gossip from mere thoughtlessness rather than to gratify ill-natured feeling. A patient ought to be able to look to his nurse as his best friend for the time being, and to feel that everything concerning his most private life is as safe with her as with himself.

The Fee for Nursing

The charge made for a nurse varies somewhat in different town and districts. For many years there was a uniform fee of a guinea a week, but of late the price has risen, and it is no uncommon thing to be asked two or even three guineas.

The institutions charge extra for surgical cases, for fever cases, for mental cases, for cases of influenza, and in fact for almost any disease that a patient is likely to suffer from. No one objects to pay an extra fee in cases of fever, for the nurse runs an extra risk, and has to go into quarantine for a time, but why an additional charge should be made because the patient is attended by a surgeon, and has to undergo some trifling operation, is not very clear.

It will be remembered that the fee is not the only expense, for the nurse must be fed, and will expect an allowance for washing as well as for cab fares and travelling expenses. If the money actually went into the pocket of the nurse it would not be grudged, but as the nurse, as a rule, receives a salary of £25 or £30 a year, or less, there seems to be no particular reason for giving her three guineas a week. There are in some towns co-operative nurses' associations, which pay over to the nurse the whole of the fee minus seven and a half percent for working expenses. These associations are popular with nurses and attract the skilled hands. It is usually perfectly safe to deal with them, for it is to their interest to send out only competent people.

Patients at the conclusion of a long illness often ask the doctor if they are expected to make the nurse a present. The answer is decidedly in the negative, the patient pays the full fee for her services, and if she is underpaid by the institution from which she is obtained, he can hardly be expected to make up the deficiency. It may happen, however, that the nurse has been exceptionally kind and attentive, and that the patient is really desirous of giving her some little memento, something that will convey to her in a tangible form his appreciation of her services. There can, of course be no possible objection to this. It may be contrary to the rules of the institution, but the patient is not bound by them. He had better take care that the present to the nurse assumes a form that will be personally useful to her, and he must give her to understand that it is for her use and hers alone, and that it is not to be handed over to the nursing home.

The Choice of a Sick Room

Much of the comfort and peace of mind of a patient during a protracted illness depends on the careful selection of a room in which to be ill. The ordinary sleeping apartment may be quite unsuited for the purpose. It is often a good plan to convert the sitting-room into the sick-chamber. The room should, if possible, face the south, so that the sun may shine in freely. If the patient has the misfortune to be in a room with a north aspect the sooner a change is made the better. It is essential to turn out all unnecessary furniture, and the carpet must be taken up. There must, of course, be a fireplace in the room, not only for the purposes of warmth, but to ensure efficient ventilation. It is convenient to have two rooms, either communicating by folding doors, or at all events adjacent. A screen is handy for keeping off draughts, especially in the winter.

The sick-room should be a large one, not only because the patient never leaves it night or day, but because the air of it is consumed by his nurses and other attendants, besides himself. Directly a patient is well enough to be left alone at night, he should be so left, because the air of a room occupied by one person will keep fresher than when occupied by two. Excepting when a person is very seriously and acutely ill, it is always advisable that the night nurse should remain in an adjoining room rather than in the sick-room, provided that the patient has ready and certain means of communicating with her.

Ventilation

One of the first essentials in a sick-room is efficient ventilation. If the room is not well-ventilated the patient will make no progress. A sick-room ought always to be so fresh that a person coming from the outside should be unable to recognise any feeling of closeness or any improper smell, but a nurse should be taught that when an open window is impossible, either from the state of the weather or the condition of the patient, that there are ways of ventilating a room without creating a draught.

If the bottom sash of the window be pulled a little upwards, and a piece of board or a sandbag be inserted between the bottom of the sash and the sill, the air will enter at the opening left between the junction of the two sashes, and the incoming current will travel upwards to the ceiling, and not laterally in anyway. In this way there will be a constant renewal of the air, but no draught will be possible.

A careful nurse will always be on her guard, not only to admit fresh air from without, but also to keep the air of the room as pure as possible. Nothing that can foul the air should be allowed to remain in the room longer than is absolutely necessary. All the excretions of the patient are to be removed with as little delay as possible. No cooking is to be carried on if it can be avoided, and all pungent cooking is to be carried on if it can be avoided, and all pungent liquids, such as brandy, wine, or medicine, should be kept in some adjoining room.

If food or stimulants be spilt upon the bedclothes, they should, if possible, be changed, for nothing is so antagonistic to appetite as the sickening smell of spilled wine, brandy, or beef tea. The room should be kept clean, and in order that it may be kept as clean as possible with the least amount of trouble, it is always advisable at the at the beginning of an illness to disencumber it as far as possible of all superfluous furniture.

Carpets, bed-hangings, heavy window curtains, wardrobes filled with wearing apparel, should be removed. A few strips of carpet by the bedside and in front of the fire give an air of comfort, and if these can be thoroughly shaken out of doors everyday there is no harm in retaining them.

The room should be thoroughly swept and dusted every day, and a good nurse will manage to effect this almost without attracting the attention of the patient. It is necessary that this should be done, and none but a bad nurse will neglect it.

Pastilles and strong scents are to be employed as little as possible, and if a room be kept clean this will be seldom necessary. A few flowers growing in pots are a cheerful addition to the sick-room, and the pleasant scent of them - if not too strong - is agreeable to the patient. Such strong-smelling flowers as hyacinth, magnolia, gardenia, or orange-blossom should not be used.

Some people have a prejudice against 'night air,' and erroneously think that it is to be excluded at any price. Such a notion arises from ignorance;

and if the windows be kept open in the manner we have directed, they may be left so throughout the whole of the night.

Light

At night time, it is advisable to burn a light, but it should be remembered that a light fouls the air of a room as much as a living being, and that the presence of a nurse and a light in a sick-room, in addition to the patient, is quite a serious tax upon its power of proper ventilation.

A night-light should be as small as possible, and should burn a very small flame. It should be looked upon rather as a means from which a proper light may be obtained in case of necessity, than as a regular source of illumination for the room. A gas-jet turned to its lowest is the best form of night-light; failing this, any of the ordinary night-lights answer the purpose admirably.

Although the daylight is not to be excluded during the day, care must be taken that it is not too obtrusive in the early morning during the summer months. It very often happens that invalids who are restless during the early hours of the night begin to fall asleep and to doze about four o'clock in the morning, and it is on all accounts important to take care that the early sunlight does not disturb the precious morning slumber.

A sick-room should not be unnecessarily darkened. It sometimes happens that an invalid cannot bear the light, or that it is desirable to encourage repose in every way, inclusive of shutting out the light, but if no good cause to the contrary exists, daylight should be freely admitted.

Daylight is cheerful, and its free admittance to every corner of a room is conducive to cleanliness. There can be little doubt also that daylight is necessary for is necessary for perfect health, and that under its influence nutrition is more active. If a sick-room be kept too dark, as very often is the case, it soon becomes very difficult for the occupant of it to bear the light at all, and he becomes markedly sensitive and delicate.

Temperature

In this country, it is almost always necessary to have a fire in a sick-room. A fire gives warmth, and it also assists ventilation very materially. The fire should be brisk with a bright flame. A sluggish fire backed up with cinders and ashes is of very little use for ventilation.

A thermometer should always be kept in a sick-room, and it should be placed as near the centre as possible. The temperature should not be lower than 60° Fahrenheit, and in many cases, especially of lung disease, it is deemed advisable to have the temperature considerably higher. A thermometer is obviously the only safe guide to temperature. The feelings of the nurse or the patient are of little use. It is very important not to let the fire go out or get too low during the night or early morning, which is the coldest time of the four-and-twenty hours. Many a patient with bronchitis has been killed by the negligence of his nurse in this respect.

Noise

It is essential that a sick-room should be quiet, but the precautions which are taken to ensure quietness are often quite unnecessary. The straw in the street and the muffled knock are the familiar insignia of sickness. Sudden starting noises are those which annoy the sick most; while, on the other hand, it is astonishing how little the patients in the London hospitals heed the inevitable noise which is incessantly going on both within and without.

Unnecessary noise, or noise that creates an expectation in the mind, is that which hurts a patient. It is rarely the loudness of the noise, the effect upon the organ of the ear itself, which appears to affect the sick. How well a patient bears the putting up of scaffolding close to the house, when he cannot bear the talking - still less the whispering - outside his door.

Never to allow a patient to be waked, intentionally or accidentally, is a *sine qua non* of all good nursing. If he is roused out of his first sleep, he is almost certain to have no more sleep. It is a curious fact, that if a patient is waked after a few hours instead of a few minutes' sleep, he is much more likely to sleep again.

Pain, like irritability of brain, perpetuates and intensifies itself. If you have gained a respite of either in sleep, you have gained more than the mere respite. Both the probability of recurrence, and of the same in intensity, will be diminished; and both will be increased by want of sleep. This, too, is the reason why a patient waked in the early part of his sleep loses, not only his sleep, but his power to sleep. A healthy person who allows himself to sleep during the day will lose his sleep at night. But it is exactly the reverse with the sick; the more they sleep, the better they are able to sleep.

It is important never to allow one's self to indulge in conversation in a sick-room in which a patient cannot, or is not meant to, participate. Although noise is to be avoided as much as possible, it must be remembered that a certain amount of work *must* be done, and that the performing of it will entail a certain amount of noise.

A good nurse will thoroughly make up her mind as to what is necessary to be done, and then, being fully satisfied as to the necessity of action – be it the making up of the fire, the cleaning of the room, the administration of food or medicine, or what not – she will set about her work and perform it thoroughly, quickly, and with the least amount of noise that is consistent with thoroughness.

An inexperienced nurse will take ten minutes to poke the fire, moving one coal at a time, and inserting the poker between the bars with absurd gentleness. In the end, the fire is not properly made up, the patient is bothered beyond expression by the persistent fidgeting, or perhaps wakes with a start as a big knob of coal falls with a crash into the fender. For merely replenishing the fire, knobs of coal may be placed upon it with the gloved hand; but it is better to make it up thoroughly, and run the risk of half a minutes noise, than to keep up an undercurrent of disturbance for a quarter of an hour.

General Rules

It is important for a nurse to fully recognize the fact that she cannot always be with her patient. It is greatly to the advantage of the patient that the nurse should keep in good health and it is incumbent upon her to arrange for proper rest, and for a due amount of exercise.

In making these arrangements, however, she must be careful to place someone in charge during her absence, and to see that the person in charge is duly instructed as to the proper course to pursue. It is during the absence of the nurse that injudicious visits are often paid to patients, and that they become tired out by conversation. A good nurse will always foresee the possibility of the little *contretemps*, and will guard against them.

Some nurses fail to realise what it is to be in charge. To be in charge is not only to carry out the proper measures yourself, but to see that everyone else does so too; to see that no one either wilfully or ignorantly thwarts or prevents such measures. It is neither to do everything yourself nor to appoint a number of people to each duty, but to ensure that each does the duty to which he or she is appointed. This is the meaning which must be attached to the word by those in charge of patients, whether of numbers or of individuals. One sick person is often waited on by four with less precision, and is really less cared for, than those who are waited on by one.

A nurse should never suggest any alteration of treatment without first consulting the medical man in charge. By so doing she may cause much disappointment to the patient, and may loosen that confidence which ought, in the patient's interest, to exist between her and the doctor. A doctor is always glad to receive any suggestion, or hear any proposition made by a nurse.

Anon, 1895

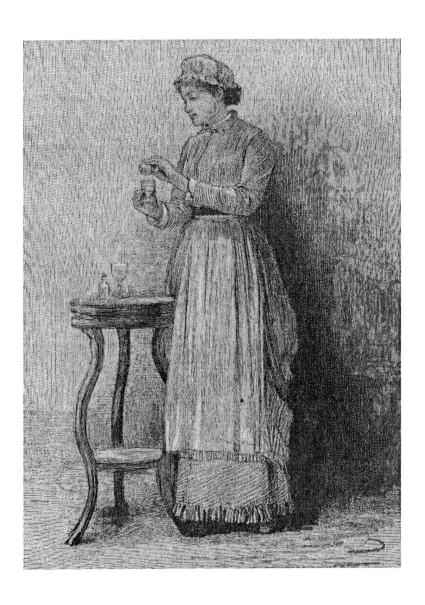

The Nurse

APPENDIX

A Great Charity Reform

The pedestrian making his way along the broad sidewalks of Fourteenth street between Broadway and Fifth Avenue, in New York City, thronged with well-dressed women eagerly bent on shopping errands, would scarcely notice, in the midst of the Parisian glitter of gilt signs which cover the fronts of the buildings, a modest tablet with the inscription 'State Charities Aid Association.'

If however, it should strike his eye, and curiosity or a real interest in charitable work should lead him to climb two pairs of stairs in search of the offices of the Association, he would find two light, large, airy rooms, tenanted by two or three serious, kind-faced ladies busily engaged writing amid piles of books, pamphlets, and letters. These ladies look as if they had found a work in life worth doing, and were doing it with all their might. The visitor would not imagine, however, unless he were informed beforehand of the character of this work, that it is one of the most far-reaching, practical, and successful efforts of genuine benevolence to be found in the United States - an effort admirable in principle, method, and details, carried on persistently year after year, ever-widening in its scope, and throwing off from itself like planets from a central sun many independent forms of kindred philanthropy.

These ladies represent an organization that is grappling with the whole vast problem of pauperism in the City and State of New York, that has branches in thirty-two of the counties of the State, and that sends its visiting committees into the poorhouses, almshouses, asylums, and hospitals to bring the eye and conscience of public opinions to bear to secure needed reforms, to elevate and moralize the whole system of relieving poverty, to send comfort to the bedsides of the destitute sick, and to instruct and interest all who have charge of sick or well in the best methods of preventing and curing the great social disease of pauperism.

The underlying idea of this comprehensive scheme of charitable work is, that all public intuitions are almost sure to generate abuses, or at least to fall into routine ways that become almost as bad as abuses, and that to keep them up to a high standard of efficiency and open to the reception of improved methods, the constant watchfulness of enthusiastic, zealous, voluntary supervision is needed.

The labors of the sanitary and Christian commissions during the war enforced this lesson, and it was to some extent the example of their labors which led to the establishment of the State Charities Aid Association.

What was the origin of this peculiar society, which has no prototype, but is evidently destined to serve as a model for like organizations in other States? Its plan grew out of the thoughts, experiences, and benevolent purpose of one woman. Earnest helpers, men and women, were found to aid in putting the plan in practice, but the conception of the scheme is due to Miss Louisa Lee Schuyler.

About ten years ago, Miss Schuyler visited the poorhouse of Westchester County, not far from her home. She was shocked at the condition of the institution. Sick and well, sane and demented, adults and children, the vicious and the merely unfortunate were huddled together, without proper sanitary conditions, or decent separation of the sexes, or any reformatory opportunities.

She took hold of the work of renovating this institution, associated with her a number of ladies living in the neighborhood, and in the course of a few months accomplished a remarkable reform. While engaged in this effort, she was impressed with the thought that, to have a permanent effect, the sort of work she was doing must not be casual and intermittent nor regular and systematic. If vigilance were relaxed, old abuses or new ones would be sure to gain a foothold. Here was struck the key-note of the great plan of benevolence which she subsequently founded.

A permanent visiting committee was formed to keep a constant oversight on the Westchester poorhouse, and this committee became the model for the committees afterward started in other counties by the central society, which was soon to come into being. Early in 1872 the Central Society was established, and received the name of the State Charities Aid Association.

Its objects, as set forth in its constitution, were:

'1st. To promote an active interest in the New York State institutions of public charities, with a view to the physical, mental, and moral improvement of the pauper inmates;

'2nd. To make the present pauper system more efficient, and to bring about such reforms in it as may be in accordance with the most enlightened views of Christianity, science, and philanthropy.'

The first president was Professor Theodore W. Dwight; Miss Schuyler was vice-president, and Miss R. B. Long, secretary. Three committees on children, on adult able-bodied paupers, and on hospitals were formed, to which was subsequently added a committee for the elevation of the poor in their homes.

Leading clergymen, physicians, and ladies of high social standing, well known for their philanthropic labors, took an interest in the movement. The membership was enlarged from month to month, and before the end of the year the Association was fairly equipped to begin its arduous under-taking. Practical wisdom was shown at the outset by not trying to do too much at once.

A much-needed work of reform was found close at hand, and for a time the efforts of the Association were chiefly concentrated upon its accomplishment. The great Bellevue Hospital in the city of New York is the omnium-gatherum of the waifs and dregs of society. The tramp, the drunkard, the outcast, the wanderer, and the honest workman who has fallen into destitution, when stricken by disease or prostrated by accident, are carried to its wards.

There are hospitals in the metropolis sustained by church organizations or endowed by private charity, and upon the islands in the East River there are public buildings for incurables, the insane, and the blind; but Bellevue is the general receptacle of all cases for which there is no better provision, and the sorting-place for patients on their way to other institutions.

A committee of sixty ladies and gentlemen was organized by the Association to make weekly visits to all the wards of this vast hive of stricken humanity. The work was done patiently and systematically.

A radical defect was discovered at the start in the system of nursing. The nurses were ignorant, illiterate women, often intemperate (though not criminals as formerly) and utterly untrustworthy. As a result the patients died from neglect, as well as from disease, and doctors were obliged to refrain from prescribing certain remedies and methods of treatment, because the nurses could not carry them out.

It seems incredible that the lives of sick people could have been left in such care. There was no lack of medical skill, for the physicians felt the pride of their profession; but it was not supplemented by the good nursing which is as important as good medical treatment.

How to provide efficient nurses for Bellevue and to break up the miserable system fastened upon it, was the first great problem that the Aid Association undertook to solve. One of its members, Doctor W. Gill Wylie, volunteered to go to Europe and study the methods of nursing employed in the public hospitals there. He visited London, Paris, and Vienna. It was in London that he found what he was seeking in the training-school for nurses established by Florence Nightingale.

His report on that school, and on the work its pupils do in the London Hospitals, was made the basis of immediate action by the Association. The result of this effort was the establishment of the Bellevue Hospital Training-school for Nurses.

Space is lacking here to describe the growth and workings of this admirable institution. A separate article would be required to give anything like a fair presentation of its successful labors in revolutionizing the system of nursing in the city hospitals, in bringing comfort and restored health to thousands of sufferers, and in sending abroad into the community hundreds of skillful, patient, gentle women, ready to answer the calls of private families for aid in the care of the sick.

In the second year of its existence, the presidency of the Association was accepted by Miss Schuyler by the desire of all its members, and she has held the position ever since. The roll of city members was considerably enlarged, studies of the problems of pauperism diligently prosecuted, and the visiting work extended to nearly all the institutions under the charge of the New York Commissioners of Charities and Corrections, except the prisons, which are the special care of the Prison Association -a well managed society of kindred character that has done admirable service in its peculiar field.

But the Aid Association was not content with what it was doing in the metropolis. Its original plan was to extend its watchful eyes and helping hands all over the State, and this plan it early began to put into effect. County after county was visited by officers of the Association, and branch local visiting committees were formed.

Sometimes, the reports of the work in New York City and in Westchester County stimulated a voluntary local movement, to which the central organization gave form and direction; but oftener a local interest had to be created by the efforts of Miss Schuyler and her associates. With rare exceptions, the county poorhouses were found in a wretched condition - buildings were not adapted for the purpose, there was no proper separation of inmates, children were contaminated by the vicious conversation of hardened reprobates, scanty provision was made for labor, miserable conditions for health existed, and no reformatory influences were at work, except an occasional sermon by some self-sacrificing clergyman.

The people living in the vicinity of a poorhouse were usually in total ignorance of what went on within its walls. They seemed to regard it as a sort of lazaretto to be avoided. The common opinion was that the place ought not to be made too comfortable, lest paupers should prefer to live in it to shifting for themselves. The Aid Association held a different theory. They believed in providing for paupers every necessary condition of healthful, moral living; but they had an infallible safeguard against overcrowded poorhouses, and that was hard work. 'Provide work for everyone who is able to work,' was the lesson they taught. Wherever it was heeded, the poorhouse flock was speedily thinned of its black sheep, for the lazy and shiftless preferred to earn wages elsewhere for work no harder than that which in the county institution only got them board and clothes.

In the formation of local visiting committees, the officers of the State Charities Aid Association follow a method which rarely fails of success. They invite a number of influential people of high standing to meet and talk the matter over. Thus an interest is aroused, other gatherings follow, the best plans of visiting work, the cure of the destitute sick, the character and management of the local poorhouse, methods of outdoor relief, the tramp nuisance, what can be done for pauper children, etc., are discussed, and soon an active, zealous local committee is created, strong enough to bring the public opinion of the community to bear in support of its plans or reform. The aim is always to get the best people into the movement, so as to give it character and force, and enable it to overcome official opposition.

As early in its career as 1873, the Association found the need of State authority to open the doors of the public institutions to its visitors. In a few cases admission was refused, and in others it was granted in a grudging, unfriendly way.

The Association consulted with the State Board of Charities, and a bill was prepared under which the two bodies could act harmoniously together. The bill, which was passed at the session of 1873, provided that visitors named by the State Board should at all times have the right to enter and inspect any of the State institutions. It was agreed between the Board and the Aid Association that the latter should nominate visitors, and that the former should give them the official authorization provided for by the new law. During seven years of cooperation between the two organizations, a great work was accomplished for the reform and elevation of the pauper institutions of the State.

Fruitful of wise plans of improvement, and tireless in their efforts to remedy defects and vices, the zealous members of the Association accomplished far more than any official body could possibly have effected by itself. Indeed, their achievements were mainly quite out of the line of regular official effort. One of the first great evils with which they grappled was the rearing of pauper children in poorhouses. They asserted that, in the interest of the State as well as of humanity, the children of paupers should not be allowed to grow up in the atmosphere of pauperism, to follow in the footsteps of their parents. Even with the best management, a poorhouse, they said, is no fit place for a child.

In some of these institutions, the visitors found three generations of the same pauper families. The taint of shiftlessness and dependence was no doubt in the blood, but society had done nothing to counteract it by proper education and surroundings. No self-respect nor ambition could be expected of a poorhouse child, reared among outcasts and the wrecks of dissipation and misfortune, and despised by all the children of the neighborhood.

The efforts of the State Board and of the Association, procured in 1875 the passage of an act which struck a great blow at the old poorhouse system. This act, with some subsequent amendments, removed all children over two years of age from poorhouses and alms-houses, and forbade such institutions to receive them. Some were sent to reformatories, industrial homes, and asylums; but the effort of the Association was to have them, as far as possible, placed in families. Institution life in its best phases, the Society holds, cannot equip a child for independence and an honorable career nearly so well as the training of an orderly household.

In their efforts to provide homes for pauper children, the Association has received valuable assistance from the Children's Aid Society of the City of New York - one of the noblest and most efficient of the great charities of the metropolis. The law does not execute itself, however, and the Association finds a great deal of work necessary to see that it is put in operation and kept in operation. At one of the meetings of the Association, when the subject of preventing pauperism by giving a proper training to the children of paupers was under consideration, Dr. Elisha Harris related the terrible story of 'Margaret, the Mother of Criminals.' It has been published in the newspapers, but can profitably be read again to illustrate the great importance of one branch of the Association's work.

Margaret was a pauper child left adrift in one of the villages on the upper Hudson, about ninety years ago. There was no alms-house in the place, and she was made a subject of outdoor relief receiving occasionally food and clothing from the town officials, but was never educated nor sheltered in a proper home. She became the mother of a long race of criminals and paupers, which has cursed the county ever since. The county records show two hundred of her descendants who have been criminals. In one generation of her unhappy line there were twenty children, of whom seventeen lived to maturity. Nine served terms aggregating fifty years in the State Prison for high crimes, and all the others were frequent inmates of jails and almshouses.

It is said, that of the six hundred and twenty-three descendants of this outcast girl, two hundred committed crimes which brought them upon the court records, and most of the others were idiots, drunkards, lunatics, paupers, or prostitutes. The cost to the county of this race of criminals and paupers is estimated as at least one hundred thousand dollars, taking no account of the damage they inflicted upon property and the suffering and degradation they caused in others. Who can say that all this loss and wretchedness might not have been spared the community if the poor pauper girl Margaret had been provided with a good moral home life while she was growing up to womanhood?

One of the most active and faithful of the Association's force of visitors engaged in the work of regular inspection of the work of regular inspection of the public charitable institutions of New York City was asked recently to give an account of a days visiting on the Islands. She said, in reply;

'We leave home about nine in the morning, land at the upper dock on Blackwell's Island, and go first to the alms-house. Here are in round numbers one thousand inmates. The aged, infirm, epileptic and disabled fill the wards. Do not suppose that we merely pass through the wards. We must look into everything see how the food is cooked, look at the supplies, examine the laundry, peer into nooks and corners, and talk with the officers about needed improvements.

'The sick of the alms-house are now cared for in pavilions a short distance from the main building, and thither we next bend our steps. Two of the long, low pavilions are for incurables, and in them there are usually about one hundred patients, men and women in about equal numbers, most of them old and suffering from diseases accompanying old age. For these poor creatures there is no real relief until death comes.

'Next in our tour comes the Insane Asylum for women. This week there are 1,270 inmates. A careful observer would notice at once the cheerless, dreary look of the corridors where the patients pass their time, the white walls, the utter absence of any bright colors, the lack of pleasant occupation. One might readily think the asylum a prison and the inmates prisoners. When they go out for an airing they go in groups, all clad alike, and move along at an even pace like so many automatons. The dull, monotonous, humdrum existence must have a depressing effect.

'The Retreat is a most melancholy place. The violent insane are kept here like so many animals behind bolts and bars.

'The next institution we visit is the Workhouse. This is another massive structure, very like a prison. The building is of stone and was built by convict labor. The cells open out on the balconies. In each cell there are two bunks -iron frames with canvass laced upon them. A single blanket is allowed to each bunk. In 1879 there were 16,408 commitments to this institution—most of them for drunkenness and disorderly conduct.

'A large proportion of the inmates belong to the army of 'repeaters,' or 'revolvers,' as the persons are called, who revolve back and forth between the workhouse and their haunts in the city. Some have been here thirty or forty times. These people perform most of the hard work of the institutions as 'helpers.' The women are scrubbers, etc. The men have a tailor-shop, shoe-shop, carpenter and blacksmith shops. They also make brooms, chairs, and scrub-brushes. Much of the clothing and bedding is also made in the workhouse. The name of this institution is no misnomer; the inmates certainly work, but none too hard; the self-commitments prove this.

'The glaring fault here is the lack of proper classification. The hardened and vicious are in the constant companionship of those who come for the first time. Neither is there any system of rewards of merit to encourage good behaviour. One great need, apparent to every woman who visits the institution, is a temporary home for friendless young girls to which they could go when discharged from the workhouse. For the want of such a home, they drift back into their old vicious associations, and finally become hardened criminals. If they could be brought under good influences, in a temporary home from whence they could be sent to some employment, a large number of them would be saved.

'The workhouse has its own hospitals, which we must inspect. Then we go to the great Charity hospital, a large stone building, five stories high, on the southern end of Blackwell's Island. The separate wooden pavilions are now used as lying-in wards. But the structure on the extreme point of the island we are not allowed to enter, for there are the smallpox cases.

'The day is not yet gone, and we take a boat for Randall's Island, where there is a frightful aggregate of human suffering. Not only the insane and the idiots are there, but the insane idiots perfect monstrosities of mental deformity. But strange to say, even these distressed creatures have a spark of harmony in their warped beings. Last Sunday they tried to sing and appeared to enjoy it when the missionary sang some hymns to them. They know enough to dress themselves and take their own seats at table, and to notice strangers. The brightest of the idiots go to school, and some of them are docile and behave themselves very well.

'A visit to the hundreds of poor sick and deformed children is touching enough. These suffering waifs appeal strongly to our sympathy. The one redeeming feature is that those who are able go to school. The buildings for the children ought to be enlarged, and everywhere better nurses are needed.

'The Branch Charity Hospital on Randall's Island receives the surplus of the other Institutions, which are generally incurable cases. The sun is getting low now, but we have still another institution to visit: the Infants Hospital for orphan babes and for mothers from the workhouse with young infants.

'In a recent year, 180 of these women were sent here by the

Superintendent of the Out-Door Poor, and 780 children were admitted, of whom 362 were orphans and 113 foundlings. You may imagine that we find enough to do in looking after the welfare of all these poor waifs. Harts and Wards Islands are also under the supervision of our Association, but they do not come within my visiting range.

'I have sought only to give you a sketch of a day's tour of a member of one of our visiting committees. It is dark when we return to the city, tired out in mind and body, but comforted for all the dreadful sights of misery, suffering, and vice we have seen with the thought that we are doing something, however little, to lessen the appalling sum of human wretchedness.'

How great the field of labor is in which the State Charities Aid Association engages in the single direction of poorhouse and alms-house inspection and reform, will be understood by a few figures from the official statistics. In 1880 there were relieved in these institutions 137,777 persons, including more than 5,000 insane. The estimated value of the aggregate property was $6, 000, 000, and the expenditures for the year $2,300,000. There is another wide field in which the Association engages with intelligence and zeal - that of curing the tramp evil and improving local methods of outdoor relief.

Some startling exposures were made a few years ago by the committee of the Association on adult able-bodied paupers, of which Mr. George H. Forster was chairman. The reports of the visiting committees in many of the rural and suburban counties showed that the overseers of the poor were interested in entertaining as large a number of tramps as possible, as they made a profit on their board and lodging. Some of these overseers were paid at the rate of one dollar for two meals and a lodging for each tramp accommodated over night. Others were paid twenty-five cents a meal, on which they probably made a profit of ten or fifteen cents.

Each overseer's house became a center of pauperism and vagrancy, and it was natural that the overseer should treat his boarders well so that they would stop at his place again. In short, he was a tramp's landlord, keeping a free hotel for vagrants at the expense of the county. The community, under this system, said in effect to the idle and vicious:

'We will board you free of cost if you will only come and stay among us.'

As a result of these exposures, the Tramp Act of 1880, drafted by the Association, was passed by the Legislature, which punishes 'tramping' with imprisonment at hard labor. Its effects have thus far been excellent. The leading idea of the Association in all its plans for dealing with able-bodied pauperism is to make the paupers work for their victuals and lodging. The same method that empties the poorhouses of half their inmates clears the roads of the stout and impudent beggars who start out to force society to give them an unearned living.

'Make them work, insists the Association, even if their labor is unprofitable to the town. Set them to breaking stone or carting dirt on the highways—anything that will show them they cannot subsist upon the community without giving some equivalent in muscular exertion.' Towns and counties that strictly follow this plan are soon shunned by the tramps, and enjoy a delightful immunity from this pest developed by careless habits of indiscriminate charity. The conclusions reached by the Association on the subject of outdoor relief, after years of study and investigation, will perhaps surprise those who think that generous giving is genuine charity. The members of the Association believe that there is too much, instead of too little, of this form of benevolence —that a vast amount of money is wasted, and a deal of evil done, by undermining the self-respect of recipients, fostering a spirit of dependence opposed to self-support, and interfering with the laws which govern wages and labor.

In New York City, there are more than sixty societies engaged in giving outdoor relief to the poor, and besides almost every church goes to some extent into the same work. In a great city, a considerable amount of such relief must be given to keep the unfortunate from suffering and death; but the Association urges that it should be given systematically and carefully, and only after a special investigation of the circumstances of each case. The motive, after relieving the most pressing necessity, should always be to help the poor to help themselves, and they should not be allowed to get into the way of thinking that whenever their affairs come to a tight pinch there is always a charitable society to fall back upon.

A large number of families are kept constantly in the borderland between self-support and pauperism, passing frequently from one region to the other, by the ease with which they can obtain money, clothes, and food from charitable societies when they are in a strait; whereas, if aid were not so convenient to obtain, they would outgrow their shiftless habits and become permanently self-sustaining. Good results are anticipated through the recent establishment of the Charity Organization Society of New York. Cooperation of all the organized charities of the city and central supervision is the plan of this society, and it is already realized to an important extent.

About four years ago an active member of the Association, Miss Sarah T. Sands, basing her work upon one of the publications of the Association, formed the Loan Relief Association, of the Sixteenth Ward, the object of which is to lend to the worthy poor small sums of money to meet pressing temporary needs, and articles required in the care of the sick - money and articles to be promptly returned at the times agreed upon.

The success of this modest little work of benevolence has been very gratifying. The Society provides medical treatment for the sick and legal assistance to people who do not know their rights or cannot hire a lawyer to lay their grievances before a court. It has a small circulating library, and a system of giving out sewing to poor women to enable them to repay with work the money they borrow. Its work has shown that as keen a sense of honor may be found in the tenement house as in the Fifth Avenue mansion. The care taken of borrowed articles, and the effort made to return money loans on the day promised, shows an integrity of character too often wanting in the rich.

One of the admirable features of the Loan Relief Society is the small expense attending it. The office of the Society is in the basement of the manager's house, so no rent is paid; nor are there any salaries to officers. The efforts of the Committee on the Elevation of the Poor in their Homes, which has in charge one of the most important branches of the permanent work of the State Charities Aid Association, deserves special notice. The chairman is Miss Grace H. Dodge. A movement in favor of tenement house reform was started by this Committee in 1879.

Important amendments to the Tenement-House Act were, in consequence, passed by the Legislature, which have brought about great improvements in the sanitary condition of the homes of the poor in the metropolis. Increased power and additional funds were given the Board of Health as a result, in part, of the agitation set on foot by the Committee. A pamphlet was printed for the use of the visitors of the Association, to enable them to instruct the dwellers in tenements as to their rights under the law in the matter of sanitary appliances required to be provided by landlords. Out of the general movement initiated by the Association and the widespread interest excited by several public meetings, grew the Improved Dwellings Association, of which Mr. W. Bayard Cutting is president - a commercial enterprise based on a humanitarian motive - and the Sanitary Reform Society, Mr. James Gallatin, president, which co-operates with the Health Department in securing the enforcement of the Health Laws.

'One good turn deserves another,' says the old proverb. One good effort stimulates another, is the experience of the Association. In the broad field of the humanities there is always enough to do, and every good work undertaken seems to open the way to others that are only waiting for earnest hands.

In 1880, the Aid Association was, by the unexpected action of the State Board of Charities, placed in a position where its usefulness would have been seriously crippled, if not destroyed, had it not speedily found a way of extricating itself. The two bodies, the official and the volunteer, had been working in harmony, as we have seen, the Association furnishing and instructing committees of visitors to the public institutions, and the Board arming them with its mandate for admission.

The system was not a good one, but its defect was not strikingly manifested until it had existed for nearly seven years, when the essential differences between the methods of volunteer workers and those of officials, was brought home to the Board by the publications in the newspapers by members of the Association of facts relating to the management of public institutions of charity. Thereupon the Board adopted rules for visitors receiving its legal appointments, which made all information obtained by the visitors the exclusive property of the Board, and not to be submitted elsewhere without its consent. This was in effect to tell the committees formed by the faithful and intelligent efforts of the Aid Association that they could not report directly to the body to which they belonged, nor act under its guidance.

Thus the whole system of volunteer inspection was threatened with destruction. The Association went to the Legislature for relief, but could accomplish nothing the first winter, the State Board of Charities being opposed to their bill. During the session of 1881 the effort was renewed. Devoted members of the central organization and of the local visiting committees went to Albany; a leading lawyer of New York, Mr. Joseph H.

Choate, gave his services, and made a convincing argument before the committee having the subject in charge; the powerful city newspapers took up the cause of the volunteers, and finally, after a great deal of effort a bill was passed authorizing judges of the Supreme Court, on the application of the managers of the State Charities Aid Association, to give authority to such persons as might be designated in such applications to visit and inspect the poorhouses and alms-houses in the counties where the visitors were residing.

It was a great victory for the principles upon which volunteer inspection is based. It gave the Association an independent legal standing, greatly encouraged its members, by removing what seemed to be an insuperable obstacle from its path, and placed its future growth and usefulness beyond peril. It should be said here that the Association fully appreciates the great value of the labors of the State Board of Charities. It insists, however, that official work in the institutions of charity needs to be supplemented by untiring volunteer effort.

An excellent result of the joint efforts of the State Board and the Aid Association may properly be mentioned here. The law of last winter establishing a State reformatory for women was urged upon the Legislature by a member of the Board, and supported by petitions circulated for signatures by the local visiting committees of the Association. This measure is exactly in line with the Association's ideas. Society, it holds, should counteract the first open signs of a tendency toward crime and degradation. Prisons too often confirm criminal instincts; 'reformatories,'' refuges,' and 'homes,' may eradicate them. Now that the Association has its own legal rights, and its own definite field of labor, it is believed a more cordial cooperation than ever will exist between its managers and the members of the State Board of Charities.

There are other interesting features of the Association's work which can only be briefly mentioned here. Who has not noticed, on coming to

New York by rail or ferry, the capacious boxes in the depots and ferry-houses, bearing a modest request for old newspapers and magazines for the use of the sick in the hospitals; and who has not felt, as he emptied his pockets of half-read dailies and periodicals, a thrill of pleasure in the thought that he was giving some poor patient, prostrated by cruel accident or lingering disease, an hours respite from the sense of his misfortune. Every day the boxes are emptied by paid agents, who distribute their contents in the hospitals.

This admirable little philanthropic plan, which does its good work as steadily and regularly as a clock, was devised by an invalid lady, and superintended by her from her sick room; at her death a fund was contributed by her friends to perpetuate the work in her memory. Books sent to the Committee on Books and Papers are distributed to public institutions through the Express Companies, free of charge. The Hospital Committees, of which Dr. Stephen Smith is chairman, and Mr. F. R. Jones is secretary, issues instructions to hospital visitors, and studies plans for hospital construction and systems of nursing and diet.

The Bellevue Training-School for Nurses, as we have already seen, grew out of its efforts. It also accomplished the important reform of removing the maternity service from the old hospital wards of Bellevue. It is consulted about the erection of new hospitals in this and other States. In regard to hospital buildings, it insists on the separate pavilion plan, believing that large, permanent structures become lurking-places for the germs of disease. Its efforts have already largely influenced public opinion in this direction.

The Association has a valuable library of American and foreign books bearing upon its various lines of work, which are loaned to its members, and to the officers of charitable institutions. Any member of a local visiting committee, or any hospital physician, can procure books by paying the postage for sending and returning. A number of pamphlets have been published by the Association to meet special needs for information. The annual reports of the Association are also a mine of good and suggestive material, available to all who desire to engage intelligently in charitable work among the poor.

The future career of the State Charities Aid Association may be outlined from its past. It proposes to maintain and strengthen its central organization, for the study of the problems of pauperism, and as a focus of thought and practical effort for the improvement of the charitable institutions and the elevation of the poorer classes, and at the same time to extend its visiting system until it embraces all the counties in the State, and brings under its inspection all the county poorhouses, city almshouses, public hospitals, and asylums.

It hopes that its success in New York will tend to the early establishment of kindred societies in other States, and is ready to assist in the organization of such societies, and give them the advantage of its experience.

Its plan of uniting the student element and the practical element in philanthropic work, by a double organization of central committees of research and visiting committees for diligent systematic work, is unique.

Nothing like it is to be found in this or any other country, and it is attracting much attention from philanthropists in England. Its managers attribute its success to the excellence of this plan, to the association of ladies and gentlemen upon all the committees, to the classification of work - not by institutions, but by persons - and to the high character and genuine benevolent spirit of those who have formed the central and local committees.

In conclusion, it should be said that the managers of the Association believe that the most urgent reform now needed in all the charitable institutions is a civil-service system, to secure a permanent tenure to meritorious officers and employees and put a stop to the vicious custom of appointments as a reward for political service. Nowhere else is there more need of experience, and of special natural fitness of character and mind, in those occupying public positions. Yet physicians, superintendents, nurses, and assistants, as a rule owe their places to their party services, or to the efforts of influential politicians, rather than to their own merit.

This wretched system is not peculiar to New York. In Ohio, not many years ago, when supremacy passed for a time from the hands of one party to that of its rival, the entire personnel of the State benevolent institutions, from superintendents down to scrubbers, was ruthlessly changed, with brutal disregard of the welfare of the unfortunate inmates. Indeed, there are few States where the offices in such institutions are not treated as the legitimate spoils of the successful party. The State Charities Aid Association, through its corps of visitors, is constantly brought in contact with the evils that grow out of this system, and will spare no effort to develop such an enlightened public opinion as will reform it altogether.

E.V Smalley, 1882

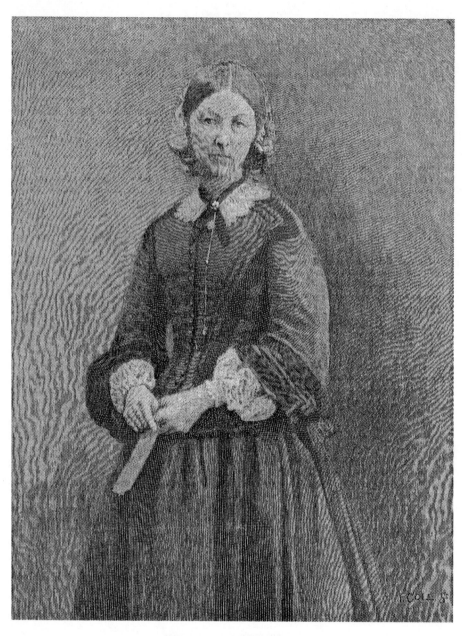

Florence Nightingale

Printed in the United States
40668LVS00006B/394